The Effective Management of Cancer Pain

Second edition

Edited by

Richard Hillier MD FRCP

*Immediate Past Chairman, Association of Palliative Medicine of Great Britain
and Ireland and Consultant in Palliative Medicine,
Southampton University Hospitals, Southampton, UK*

Ilora Finlay FRCP FRCGP

*Professor of Palliative Medicine, University of Wales College of Medicine,
Cardiff and Past Chairman, Association of Palliative Medicine of
Great Britain and Ireland, UK*

Andrew Miles MSc MPhil PhD

*Professor of Public Health Policy and UK Key Advances Series Organiser,
University of East London, UK*

UeL University Centre for
Public Health Policy &
Health Services Research

Association of Palliative
Medicine of Great Britain
and Irleand

AESCULAPIUS MEDICAL PRESS
LONDON SAN FRANCISCO SYDNEY

Published by

Aesculapius Medical Press (London, San Francisco, Sydney)
Centre for Public Health Policy and Health Services Research
School of Health Sciences
University of East London
33 Shore Road, London E9 7TA, UK

British Library Cataloguing in Publication Data
A catalogue record for this book is available from the British Library

ISBN 1 903044 21 9

While the advice and information in this book are believed to be true and accurate at the
time of going to press, neither the authors nor the publishers nor the sponsoring institutions
can accept any legal responsibility or liability for any errors or omissions that may be made.
In particular (but without limiting the generality of the preceding disclaimer) every effort
has been made to check drug usages; however, it is possible that errors have been missed.
Furthermore, dosage schedules are constantly being revised and new side effects recognised.
For these reasons, the reader is strongly urged to consult the drug companies' printed
instructions before administering any of the drugs recommended in this book.

Further copies of this volume are available from:

Claudio Melchiorri
Research Dissemination Fellow
Centre for Public Health Policy and Health Services Research
School of Health Sciences
University of East London
33 Shore Road, London E9 7TA, UK

Fax: 020 8525 8661
email: claudio@keyadvances4.demon.co.uk

Typeset, printed and bound in Britain
Peter Powell Origination & Print Limited

Contents

Contributors

Sam Hjelmeland Ahmedzai MD FRCP, Professor of Palliative Medicine, University of Sheffield

Claire Bates MA MB BS DRCOG MRCP, Specialist Registrar in Palliative Medicine, St Joseph's Hospice, London

Mike Bennett MD MRCP, Consultant in Palliative Medicine, St Gemma's Hospice, Leeds

Mary Brennan FRCP, Specialist Registrar in Palliative Medicine, Palliative Care Centre, Camden and Islington Community NHS Trust, London

Andrew Davies MB BS MSc MD MRCP, McAlpine Macmillan Consultant Lecturer in Palliative Medicine, Department of Palliative Medicine, Bristol Oncology Centre, Bristol

Rob George MA MD FRCP, Consultant in Palliative Medicine and Clinical Director, Palliative Care Centre, Camden and Islington Community NHS Trust, London

Colin Hardman MPharm MRPharmS MCPP, Senior Pharmacist, Pharmacy Department, Lincoln County Hospital, Lincoln

Richard Hillier MD FRCP, Consultant in Palliative Medicine, Southampton University Hospitals NHS Trust, and Immediate Past Chairman, Association of Palliative Medicine of Great Britain and Ireland

Anne Lanceley RGN DipN PGDE PhD, Senior Lecturer and Head of Postgraduate Studies, Centre for Cancer and Palliative Care Studies, Institute of Cancer Research, The Royal Marsden Hospital, London

Matthew K Makin MB ChB MA MRCP, Consultant in Palliative Medicine, North East Wales NHS Trust and Medical Director, Nightingale House Hospice, Wrexham, Wales

Anne Naysmith FRCP, Consultant in Palliative Medicine, Pembridge Palliative Care Centre, St Charles Hospital, London

Jennifer Smith MB MRCP, Specialist Registrar in Palliative Medicine, Mersey Deanery

Peter Speck MA BSc, Chaplaincy Team Leader, Southampton University Hospitals NHS Trust, Southampton

Teresa Tate FRCP FRCR, Consultant in Palliative Medicine, St Bartholomew's Hospital and Medical Adviser, Marie Curie Cancer Care, London

Keri Thomas MB BS DRCOG MRCGP DipPallMed, Macmillan GP Facilitator in Cancer and Palliative Care, Macmillan Adviser for the Northern Region, Calderdale and Kirklees Health Authority, Huddersfield

Catherine E Urch BSc BM MRCP, Clinical Research Fellow, Department of Pharmacology, University College London

Bee Wee MB BCh MCGP(I), Senior Lecturer and Consultant in Palliative Medicine, and Deputy Director of Education, School of Medicine, Southampton University Hospitals NHS Trust, Southampton

Giovambattista Zeppetella BSc MB MRCGP, Consultant in Palliative Medicine and Deputy Medical Director, St Joseph's Hospice, and Honorary Consultant, Barts and the London NHS Trust, London

Preface

Although the efficacy of topical opioids in the management of pain was noted as far back as the eighteenth century, it is only in the last 10 years that intense interest has focused on the expression and clinical relevance of peripheral opioid receptors. It is now established that opioids exert an anti-nociceptive effect not only by their actions on the central nervous system, but also through their effects on the peripheral nervous system. This observation has obvious implications for the management of cancer-related pain. Part 1 of the current volume reviews current perspectives in the role of peripheral opioid receptors and discusses their relevance in relation to the generation and management of cancer pain.

Cancer pain, in common with all types of pain, is essentially a subjective phenomenon and the assessment and measurement of pain should ideally be based on information provided by the patient rather than by proxies such as partners, family members and other non-professional carers whose assessments, although helpful, are rarely sufficient to inform treatment decisions. Indeed, the assessment of pain primarily depends on basic clinical skills and there are now a number of validated tools for the assessment of pain and its relief; these are becoming an increasingly important component of routine clinical practice within palliative care. Although such tools are useful in making treatment decisions, the individual's experience of pain and the success of intervention are greatly affected by a variety of factors. These may enable them to cope with pain and/or exacerbate its experience. These factors include cultural, social, psychological, emotional or spiritual factors. When all or most are involved, this contributes to so-called 'total pain'. The good clinician always listens to the patient's story, rather than relying on his or her own understanding of what it 'ought to be' – a real clinical skill that will take time to acquire and develop. Part 2 of this volume, through Chapters 2 and 3, reviews current progress in, and understanding of, the means of assessment of both physical and 'non-physical' pain.

The World Health Organization (WHO) recommends morphine as the opioid of choice for the management of moderate-to-severe cancer pain, and the dose of morphine is classically titrated against the pain to achieve analgesia. There is not thought to be a ceiling dose to the analgesic effects of morphine, although for some patients there may come a stage where a further escalation of dose risks unacceptable toxicity. It has been suggested that, for these patients, a different opioid may prove beneficial; the decision to change medication has become known as 'opioid switching'. The practice is not without its critics and much of the present evidence supporting its use derives largely from case reports and retrospective studies. These examine the practice itself and also describe a variable relationship in the equianalgesic doses between the opioids used. Chapter 4, the first chapter in Part 3, provides an insightful overview of current thinking on opioid switching, showing that prospective studies are urgently needed to make the practice more rigorously evidence based than at present.

Not all pain responds to opioids and non-opioids. In providing guidance of the management of cancer pain, the WHO considers adjuvant analgesia as an important strategy in the overall management of this symptom, with co-analgesics being particularly useful in neuropathic, bone or visceral pain unresponsive, or only partially responsive, to opioids or non-opioid analgesia. Although useful data have accumulated on the place in routine clinical practice of antidepressants, anticonvulsants, N-methyl-D-aspartate antagonists and bisphosphonates, the use of these agents in cancer pain syndromes compared with non-malignant pain syndromes is largely guided by personal experience. There remains a paucity of data from, for example, systematic reviews and meta-analyses which could assist in providing a more definitive evidence base. This fact has led to a lack of consensus. Local guidelines, have often been developed, but rarely widely, and they often advocate agents for general use before their effectiveness has been reasonably established. As with opioid switching, there is an urgent need to concentrate research effort in adjuvant analgesia on well-designed collaborative trials, which will specifically address the gaps in knowledge that are currently all too apparent within this particular area of clinical practice. Chapter 5 reviews adjuvant analgesia and Chapter 6 reviews the place of currently 'off-licence' agents, completing Part 3.

The significant variation in decision-making of cancer pain management is illustrated and discussed, using pertinent examples, in Part 3. This argues for the use of nationally or internationally agreed clinical practice guidelines. The concept of using guidelines to direct practice is not new. Their advantages and disadvantages in the context of clinical practice were discussed, for example, by Plato in the fourth century BC, who noted the tension between the voluntary nature of guidelines and the expectation that, in time, adherence to them would become mandatory, removing the physician's ability to respond uniquely to individual clinical situations. Support for the evolution of evidence-based clinical practice guidelines in palliative care has increased significantly over recent years and Chapter 7, which starts Part 4, compares and contrasts the recommendations of four sets of guidelines for the management of cancer pain within an overall discussion of the utility of practice guidelines in the process of patient care. Guidelines may enhance the quality of patient care by codifying knowledge into specific clinical recommendations or may detract from it by reducing clinical actions to common denominators, ignoring the need to tailor care in the context of the unique experience of the individual. In time, they may, however, be shown to have a role in minimising common, or even uncommon, 'errors' and may help correct deficiencies in the organisation and delivery of the clinical service. Approximately 6.5% of hospital admissions are, after all, known to be associated with an adverse drug reaction, with one in five of these probably preventable in nature. It cannot be argued that palliative care is free from such errors or indeed from other deficiencies in service provision, and Chapter 8, the concluding chapter of Part 4, presents a stimulating review of the nature of error in clinical practice and a discussion of how error might be minimised or avoided within the context of palliative medicine.

Part 5 continues the theme of quality in clinical practice with a discussion of the clinical governance of cancer pain services, a discussion of the developments necessary in the general practice setting for effective control of cancer pain, and a review of the nature and place of nurse-led interventions as part of overall patient management. Governance is undoubtedly important in cancer pain management, but there are difficulties in implementing systematic evaluations in this care setting. Indeed, effective governance requires an evidence base on which to define good practice, but at the time of writing this is largely lacking. To improve the evidence, good clinical trials must first be designed, conducted, analysed and interpreted. An obvious outcome measure with which to evaluate quality-of-service provision will be the degree of pain control, emphasising the centrality of agreed and validated pain assessment tools and their standardised use within the service, although other outcome measures will need to be devised, validated and employed if a more comprehensive evaluation and monitoring of the effectiveness and efficiency of cancer pain management services is to be achieved. The importance of multidisciplinary team working cannot be overemphasised here, and having the right team in the right place at the right time will be crucial to effective governance of pain services; outcome measures could certainly be developed with these criteria in mind.

Naturally, education remains pivotal for the management of cancer pain. Outcome measures built around this function may also represent important tools for service evaluation and development. A working knowledge of only the basics of cancer pain management is, absolutely, no longer acceptable in palliative care. Good clinical practice requires well-developed skills in assessment, an understanding of the role of analgesics and co-analgesics and non-pharmacological interventions, an ability to explain these clearly and appropriately to patients and their families, and a sound decision-making process within an ethical framework. It is clear that a range of educational methods will be required to form and maintain such high-level clinical skills and this itself begs the question of who should teach and how appropriate teachers are supported in their role. Part 6, the concluding part, carefully considers these issues with accompanying recommendations that contribute to the ongoing debate.

In the current age, when doctors and health professionals are increasingly bombarded with clinical information, we have aimed to provide a fully current, fully referenced text which has been as succinct as possible but as comprehensive as necessary. Consultants in palliative medicine and their trainees will find it of particular use in continuing professional development and specialist training, respectively, and we advance it specifically as an excellent tool for these purposes. We anticipate, however, that nurse specialists and all those members of the multidisciplinary clinical team involved in the delivery of effective palliative care services will find it of substantial value as a reference text and we commend it enthusiastically to these colleagues especially for this purpose.

In conclusion we thank Janssen-Cilag for a grant of educational sponsorship, which helped organise a national symposium held with the Association of Palliative Medicine of Great Britain and Ireland at The Royal College of Physicians of London, at which synopses of the constituent chapters of this book were presented.

Richard Hillier MD FRCP
Ilora Finlay FRCP FRCGP
Andrew Miles MSc MPhil PhD

PART 1

Peripheral opioid receptors and cancer pain

Chapter 1

The analgesic role of peripheral opioid receptors

Catherine E Urch

Introduction

The analgesic actions of topically applied opioids was noted in the eighteenth and nineteenth centuries by Heberden and Wood. Despite this, traditional teaching became that of an exclusively central analgesic action for opioids. Although this may be the case in acute pains, peripheral actions may be revealed by tissue damage. It is only in the last decade that intense interest has focused on the expression and clinical relevance of opioid receptors on the peripheral nervous system (Stein 1991).

Peripheral opioid receptors have been shown to mediate analgesic effects when activated by either endogenous or exogenous opioids. All classes of opioid receptor – μ, δ, κ – and the novel opioid-like receptor 1 (ORL-1) (Stein 1995; Taylor & Dickenson 1998) have been demonstrated on peripheral sensory nerve terminals, and have been shown to be upregulated in inflammation (Hassan *et al.* 1993). The endogenous ligands are expressed in both circulatory immune cells and peripheral sensory nerves (PSNs) (Stein *et al.* 1997) and local endogenous or exogenous opioids can produce analgesia in the inflamed area. The opioid system appears to be one part of the extensive cross-talking that occurs between the nervous system and its mobile counterpart, the immune system, to co-ordinate the organism's defence mechanisms.

Peripheral opioid receptor expression

The dorsal root ganglia (DRGs) contain mRNA for the μ, δ and κ opioid receptors, and the recently described ORL-1 (Wick *et al.* 1994; Ji *et al.* 1995; Andoh *et al.* 1997; Zhang *et al.* 1998). All classes of opioid receptors can be demonstrated on PSN fibres and terminals in normal tissue, in both animals and humans, albeit at a low level (Stein *et al.* 1990, 1997; Coggeshall *et al.* 1997). Immunohistochemical and functional studies indicate that the opioid receptors mediating analgesia appear to be confined to the primary afferent neurons, and are not present on post-ganglionic sympathetic neurons (Schafer *et al.* 1994; Zhou *et al.* 1998; Wenk & Honda 1999). The pharmacological characteristics of the classic μ, δ and κ peripheral receptors are similar to the central opioid receptors (Hassan *et al.* 1993; Stein *et al.* 1997). The ORL-1 also appears to modulate nociception; however, as specific antagonists are not yet available, the full pharmacological characteristics have not been elucidated (Taylor & Dickenson 1998).

Activation of the μ, δ and κ receptors induces peripheral anti-nociception via reduced excitability of peripheral nerve terminals, attenuation of propagation of action potentials and inhibition of pro-nociceptive compounds. Possible mechanisms include increased potassium currents, decreased calcium currents via interactions with G proteins (G_i or G_0) and the inhibition of tetrodotoxin-resistant sodium currents (Gold & Levine 1996; Xie *et al.* 1999; Rodrigues & Duarte 2000; Samoriski & Gross 2000). Opioids also inhibit the calcium-dependent release of pro-nociceptive, pro-inflammatory compounds, such as substance P from the PSNs. Centrally, the ORL-1 acts in the same manner as the classic opioid receptors, producing inhibition via G-protein linkage and adenylyl cyclase inhibition (Vaughan & Christie 1996; Henderson & McKnight 1997; Meunier 1997). The peripheral action of the ORL-1 in normal tissue in response to exogenous nociceptin/orphanin FQ (its endogenous ligand) (Meunier *et al.* 1995) is contradictory because it leads to increased excitability of the neuron and a degree of mechanical sensitisation (Carpenter *et al.* 2000). The mechanism by which opposing actions of the same receptor ligand complex can occur has not been fully explained, although α receptors have been reported to couple both excitatory and inhibitory intracellular processes (Crain & Shen 1990).

Of note, the endogenous ligand nociceptin/orphanin FQ mRNA is not found in DRGs in normal tissue, but is present rapidly in inflamed tissue (Meunier *et al.* 1995; Andoh *et al.* 1997). This is in contrast to the endogenous ligands for the μ, δ and κ receptors which are always present within the neuron and upregulated after inflammation (Stein *et al.* 1997).

Peripheral opioid receptors in inflammation

Numerous changes occur with respect to the opioid receptors on the PSN during inflammation. Within minutes the receptors become readily detectable (rapid translocation to surface expression), more available as the perineurium is disrupted and active (G protein coupled). Over the next 24–96 hours the density of the peripheral opioid receptors increases, as a result of increased DRG production and retrograde transportation, together with sprouting of the peripheral terminals.

In early inflammation, pre-existing but possibly inactive opioid receptors may be activated by the alteration in the specific milieu of inflamed tissue (Machelska *et al.* 1999a). The low pH found in inflammation increases opioid agonist efficacy by altering the interaction between the receptor and G proteins (Selley *et al.* 1993). Furthermore, opioids attenuate the excitability of primary afferents (via inhibition or cyclic adenosine monophosphate [cAMP]) to a greater extent when the neuronal cAMP levels are raised, a common scenario in inflammation (Ingram & Williams 1994). Under normal circumstances the perineurium acts as a diffusion barrier, maintaining the homoeostasis of the peripheral afferent somatic and autonomic nerve fibres (Olsson 1990). Disruption of the perineurium can be caused by inflammation or artificially by hyperosmolar solutions (Antonijevic *et al.* 1995). This disruption allows enhanced permeability and facilitates the passage of macromolecules (including opioids) to and from the sensory neuron. The early peripheral opioid analgesia in inflammation has been shown to coincide with the perineurial disruption (Machelska *et al.* 1999a).

Studies using anti-sera against the δ and κ receptors have demonstrated little overall change in DRG mRNA. However, alteration in the distribution and expression of the opioid receptors has been seen. During inflammation the µ opioid receptors are upregulated, whereas the δ and κ ones are downregulated (Ji *et al.* 1995; Zhang *et al.* 1998). The density of opioid receptors on PSNs has increased 24–96 hours after the onset of inflammation, as well as the number of PSN terminals (sprouting) (Weihe *et al.* 1988; Hassan *et al.* 1993). This increase in receptor density could be inhibited by ligating the sciatic nerve, indicating enhanced retrograde transport of the receptors (Hassan *et al.* 1993).

An autoregulatory role for the opioid receptors located on the inner surface of the PSN membranes has been suggested (Frank & Sudha 1987). Opioid peptides produced within the PSN could in theory bind to the submembrane receptors and modulate the excitability of its own axon.

The role of the ORL-1 is worth considering separately because it appears to have unique and contradictory anti-nociceptive actions centrally (in the dorsal horn) and in the PSNs. Carpenter *et al.* (2000) examined this in a carrageenan model of inflammation. An intraplantar injection of increased doses of exogenous nociceptin was given in the inflamed or normal tissue. In both situations there was an equivalent dose-responsive increase in neuronal excitability, compared with the control. This contrasted to a dose-dependent inhibition of neuronal activity in the same experimental situation, when exogenous nociceptin was given spinally. This peripheral hyperalgesic action of exogenous nociceptin is also reported by Inoue *et al.* (1998), who suggested that it was dependent on the release of substance P. However, in contrast to this position is the finding that exogenous nociceptin reduces neurogenic inflammation (Helyes *et al.* 1997). Initially, it would appear that the new family member ORL-1 opposes the classic opioid receptor action in the periphery in inflammation, while enhancing it centrally. It should be mentioned that the action of endogenous nociceptin in inflammation is not known. Indeed from the work of Carpenter *et al.* (2000) there would appear to be little or no effect. In the experimental system, the control saline injection evoked an equivalent small response in both the inflamed and non-inflamed tissue, yet the level of endogenous nociceptin would have been elevated in the latter (Andoh *et al.* 1997).

Neuroimmune interactions of opioid peptides

There is extensive interaction between the immune system and the nervous system, modulating both pathways. These interactions are mediated by a variety of molecules including peptides (corticotrophin-releasing factor [CRF]), monoamines (adrenaline, dopamine), glucocorticoids, free radicals, cytokines (interleukins 1 and 6 [IL1, IL6] and tumour necrosis factor [TNF]) and opioid peptides (Weigent & Blalock 1997). Immunoreactive endorphins and enkephalins and low levels of dynorphin have been demonstrated in T and B lymphocytes, macrophages and monocytes within inflamed tissue. There is growing evidence that these peptides are derived from the precusors pro-opiomelanocortin (POMC), and pro-enkephalin, which have been demonstrated in the immune cells in both rodents and humans (Sharp & Linner 1993; Weisinger 1995; Stefano *et al.* 1996). The same post-translational processing enzymes (the subtilase-like pro-protein convertases) are expressed in the immune cells and central nervous system (CNS), yielding differential splicing under differing conditions (Vindrola *et al.* 1994; Salzet *et al.* 2000). In normal tissue, the POMC mRNA is about 200–400 times shorter than CNS POMC (Stein *et al.* 1997). However, in pathological conditions, such as inflammation and cancer (but not in normal tissue), full-length peripheral POMC mRNA is expressed and upregulated (Sharp & Linner 1993; Cabot *et al.* 1997).

Recent studies suggest that the predominant β-endorphin-containing lymphoctyes are memory T lymphocytes that reside in the lymph nodes. Immune cells are trafficked specifically to sites of local inflammation where the endorphins are released and the depleted T lymphocyte returns to the draining lymph node (Cabot *et al.* 1997). Immunocyte recruitment is a highly specific and directed multistep process activated by the initial damage or foreign body invasion (Butcher & Picker 1996). Leucocytes are captured on the vascular endothelium via a sequential engagement of adhesion molecules, such as L-selectin on the leukocytes and E- and P-selectin on the endothelium adjacent to the site of tissue damage/invasion (Machelska *et al.* 1999a). Once activated by chemoattractants, the level of integrins is upregulated allowing firm attachment and transmigration through the endothelium. Blockade of these adhesion molecules abolishes the peripheral opioid analgesia. Pre-treatment of rats with sodium fusidate (Fucidin – a selectin blocker) prevented the arrival of endorphin-laden lymphocytes and inhibited peripheral analgesia (Machelska *et al.* 1999a).

Immune cell activation appears to lead to enhanced proteolytic processing of endorphins, which are subsequently released locally at the site of inflammation. The endomorphin content in an inflamed paw has been shown to increase over 4 days. This represented the accumulation of endorphin-containing immune cells and increased synthesis within the cells (Cabot *et al.* 1997). Locally produced CRF and IL1 appear to be vital for endorphin release, and their respective receptors on immune cells are upregulated in inflammation (Heijnen *et al.* 1991; Mousa *et al.* 1996; Schafer *et al.* 1996). Release can be blocked in vivo by CRF antagonists and immunosuppression (Schafer *et al.* 1994, 1996), and can be enhanced by stress (rats swimming in cold water increased local analgesia in an inflamed paw) and local injection of CFR or IL1 (Stein 1995; Schafer *et al.* 1996). In vitro CFR can cause the release of endorphins from lymph node suspensions (Schafer *et al*. 1997). The release is calcium dependent and can be mimicked by a rise in extracellular calcium (Cabot *et al*. 1997).

Immunomodulation of opioid peptides

Opioid-binding sites have been demonstrated on immune cells, and binding of enkephalins and endorphins has wide-ranging immunomodulatory effects – both pro- and anti-inflammatory (Stein 1995; Sharp *et al*. 1998). Opioids enhance the inflammatory reaction via increased macrophage phagocytosis, IL1 and IL6 production (both pro-inflammatory and pro-nociceptive), IL4 production (increases B-cell immunoglobulin production) and T-cell cytotoxicity (Sizemore *et al*. 1991; Kowalski 1998; Zhong *et al*. 1998). Furthermore, extravasation of fluid (oedema) secondary to a carrageenan-induced inflammation was not found to be reduced or prevented by intraplantar injections of morphine (Perrot *et al*. 1999). κ Agonists have been shown to enhance extravasation during the early phase of the formalin response, whereas μ and δ agonists inhibited it (Hong & Abbott 1995). Others reported that the site of inflammation, together with the route and dose of morphine, was the determinant factor tipping the balance towards pro- or anti-inflammatory changes (Millan & Colpaert 1991; Earl *et al*. 1994; Walker *et al*. 1996; Wilson *et al*. 1996). Low-dose morphine has been reported to be pro-inflammatory, whereas high-dose morphine attenuates inflammation.

The weight of evidence would, however, indicate that the overall effect of opioids tends to the anti-inflammatory via neuronal and immune negative feedback mechanisms (Machelska *et al*. 1999a). Neurogenic inflammation may be attenuated via reduced tachykinin release (substance P) from the local neurons, in response to increased endorphin binding. Several authors have demonstrated that opioid agonists (κ, δ and μ) can attenuate carrageenan oedema and the vascular response to electrical or substance P-induced vasodilatation (Gyires *et al*. 1985; Russell *et al*. 1985; Green & Levine 1992; Jin *et al*. 1999; Khalil *et al*. 1999) and can be antagonised by naloxone (Green & Levine 1992). Highly selective κ agonists have a potent anti-inflammatory effect when injected locally into an inflamed paw, and reduce the severity of adjuvant arthritis in rats by 80% (Wilson *et al*. 1996; Binder & Walker 1998; Binder *et al*. 2000). Immunomodulatory effects have been demonstrated in vivo and in vitro. Exposure to opioids suppressed T-lymphocyte function, and reduced synthesis and release of cytokines (Machelska *et al*. 1999a) and, clinically, intra-articular morphine was shown to reduce the inflammatory infiltrate (Stein *et al*. 1999).

The ORL-1 has been demonstrated on immune cells, including human T and B lymphocytes (Halford & Gebhart 1995; Wick *et al*. 1995; Peluso *et al*. 1998). A corresponding production of nociceptin/orphanin FQ has been demonstrated in neurons and leucocytes (Nothacker *et al*. 1996; Inoue *et al*. 1998). As the ORL-1 and its ligand nociceptin have a similar distribution to the classic opioids, it would appear to be involved in the neuroimmunoregulation of inflammation and nociception. However, the ORL-1 has only a 60% homology to the classic opioid receptors, which may indicate that it is newer in evolutionary terms (Wick *et al.* 1994; Taylor & Dickenson 1998). Thus this receptor complex may have different, as yet unknown, peripheral functions, indicated by the apparent pro-nociceptive action of peripheral nociceptin. Further work may clarify its role in the complex world of opioid neuroimmunomodulation.

Opioids induce a profound local analgesic affect via the PSN only in inflamed tissue. The activation of immune cells induces release of endogenous opioids, which in turn modulate the immune response. Thus, the evolutionary ancient interaction between the immune and neurological systems not only mounts a specific defence response, it also induces local analgesia to control the pain in the injured tissue, thus enabling control of the injury/invasion while maintaining the organism's ability to continue functioning.

Animal models

Exogenous opioids

The activation of opioid receptors on PSNs to induce a potent analgesia has been studied under a variety of pathological animal models: neuropathic pain, visceral pain, bone damage and models of inflammation (such as carrageenan, complete Freud's adjuvant, formalin, prostaglandin or neurogenic) (Stein 1993; Machelska *et al.* 1999a). Opioid-mediated analgesia appears to be greatest in inflammatory states with little or no effect in non-inflamed tissue, for the reasons discussed above. Perrot *et al.* (1999) measured the analgesic effect of increased doses of intraplantar morphine before or after the induction of carrageenan inflammation. They found a dose-related anti-nociceptive effect of morphine, consistent with reports on the efficacy of intra-articular morphine in induced arthritis (Stein 1991; Likar *et al.* 1997). Morphine also appeared to have a pre-emptive analgesic action, which was gone by 3 hours. However, morphine did not alter paw oedema or prevent the enhanced inflammatory response to a second carrageenan injection (see previous section for discussion).

Systemic adverse effects can be avoided by the local application of small, systemically inactive doses, or by altering the biological activity of the exogenous opioid such that it cannot cross the blood–brain barrier (Barber & Gottschlich 1997; Stein *et al.* 1997). Loperamide is a μ-opioid-selective agonist, developed as an anti-diarrhoeal agent, because it does not penetrate the blood–brain barrier. Loperamide was shown to be a potent anti-hyperalgesic when administered locally in an inflamed knee joint, or post-CFA (complete Freund's adjuvant) paw inflammation in rats (DeHaven Hudkins *et al.* 1999). However, loperamide failed to exhibit anti-nociception when given orally. κ-Opioid ligands have also demonstrated potent anti-nociceptive effects. When applied together with topical capsaicin, they have been shown to inhibit capsaicin-induced allodynia (Ko *et al.* 1999) and locally administered highly selective κ agonists have been shown to have a potent, long-acting anti-nociceptive effect in CFA-induced inflammation, together with a potent anti-inflammatory effect (Machelska *et al.* 1999b). Comparison of locally injected agonists for the three classic opioid receptors (μ, κ, δ) has demonstrated that μ-opioid agonists are the most potent in inducing peripheral analgesia; however, δ and κ are also active. The anti-nociceptive action were dose dependent, stereoselective and naloxone reversible, and did not occur at equivalent systemic doses (Stein *et al.* 1989; Machelska *et al.* 1999a). However, the relative potency may depend on the nature and stage of the inflammatory reaction.

Clinical studies

Endogenous opioids

Peripheral opioid actions are of clinical interest and relevance. Opioid receptors have been identified in human DRGs and PSNs (Stein *et al.* 1996), and on lymphocytes, macrophages and mast cells (mainly β-endorphin and enkephalin) in joint synovium (Stein *et al.* 1999). There is evidence of local endogenous opioid release (Yoshino *et al.* 1992) and opioid-mediated anti-nociception in patients undergoing knee surgery. Blockade of intra-articular opioid receptors with naloxone resulted in enhanced pain and an increased requirement for supplemental analgesia (Stein *et al.* 1993). It is interesting to note that the presence of endogenous opioids in inflamed tissue does not appear to interfere with exogenous opioid analgesia (Stein *et al.* 1996).

Exogenous opioids

There is a large and ever-growing body of evidence supporting the analgesic efficacy of locally administered opioids to the site of inflammation in clinical settings (some examples are shown in Table 1.1). Studies of experimentally induced pain (heat and pressure thresholds in second-degree burns or capsaicin-induced allodynia) have demonstrated the anti-nociceptive properties of small doses (1–2 mg) of morphine when given locally at the site of injury (Moiniche *et al.* 1993; Kinnman *et al.* 1997).

A large number of studies have examined the postoperative intra-articular injection of morphine (0.5–6.0 mg), and pain responses have been recorded in numerous ways: visual analogue or numerical rating scale, supplemental analgesic requirement or time to first analgesic. Together, the results demonstrate an opioid-specific (and reversible), relatively long-acting and locally specific (no systemic effect) analgesia (for review see Stein *et al.* 1997). Studies that have shown no effect often demonstrate a lack of tissue inflammation or lack a sensitive assay (Rosseland *et al.* 1999).

Several studies report the efficacy of intra-articular opioids in chronic arthritis, with some reports of a reduced inflammatory infiltrate. Numerous other novel routes

Table 1.1 The efficacy of exogenous opioids in various clinical settings

Procedure	Effects	References
Intra-articular (i.a.) opioids	Authors report changes in VAS, time to first analgesic, total analgesic requirement	Stein et al. (1991); Lawerence et al. (1992); Joshi et al. (1993); Dalsgaard et al. (1994); Likar et al. (1995, 1999); Kalso et al. (1997)
Knee arthroscopy Postoperative Morphine i.a. – low dose (0.5–6mg), no systemic side effects	Intra-articular opioids produced enhanced analgesia, dose–response, reversible naloxone	
Fentanyl i.a. vs morphine i.a.	Fentanyl analgesia > morphine	Varkel et al. (1999)
Morphine i.a. ± LA ± NSAID	Combination better analgesia: opioid + LA + NSAID > opioid + LA > opioid alone	Khoury et al. (1992); Elhakim et al. (1999)
Preoperative opioid + LA	Equally effective as postoperative combination	Gupta et al. (1999); Gurkan et al. (1999)
Morphine i.a. vs regional anaesthesia	Equally effective	Tetzlaff et al. (1999)
Morphine i.a.	Ineffective analgesia, no change in VAS or total analgesic requirement[a]	Bjornsson et al. (1994); Laurent et al. (1994); Niemi (1994); Graham et al. (2000)
Rheumatoid arthritis: morphine i.a. vs dexamethasone i.a. vs placebo	Reduction in VAS active and rest Morphine >> dexamethasone >> placebo Reduced inflammatory infiltrate	Raja et al. (1992); Aasbo et al. (1996)

continued...

Table 1.1 The efficacy of exogenous opioids in various clinical settings *continued*

Procedure	Effects	References
Osteoarthritis: morphine i.a.	Analgesia and reduced inflammation	Likar et al. (1997); Stein et al. (1999)
Other joints: morphine i.a. after temporomandibular joint arthroscopy	No alteration in VAS or analgesic requirement	Bryant et al. (1999)
Intraperitoneal (i.p.) opioids		
Sufentanil (one side) post-partum tubal ligation	26/30 reduced VAS scores on treated side > 24 hours. No alteration in overall analgesia	Schulte Steinberg et al. (1995)
Morphine i.p. post-laparoscopic cholecystectomy	No alteration in postoperative analgesia requirements[b]	Rorarius et al. (1999)
Topical		
Dental extraction: morphine preoperative, into inflamed tooth pulp + LA block	Increased analgesia, reduced extra analgesia, reduced VAS, especially > 24 hours	Likar et al. (1998)
Cornea: morphine to abraded cornea	Increased analgesia	Peyman et al. (1994)
Skin ulcers: morphine (or diamorphine) to malignant ulcers or pressure sores	Increase analgesia, rapid onset, lasts 6–8 hours. Epidermal surface must be broken to achieve analgesia	Back & Finlay (1995); Krajnik & Zylicz (1997); Krajnik et al. (1999); Twillman et al. (1999)

This table illustrates some of the reported effects of peripherally delivered exogenous opioids. The most frequently reported clinical use of peripheral opioids is in post-knee arthroscopy with more than 50 reports.

[a]The vast majority of reports indicate an increased analgesic effect of local opioids, but those that do not were not given in inflamed knee joints. Numerous other clinical settings have demonstrated the analgesic efficacy of peripheral opioids, although not all.

[b]In one intraperitoneal study no effect was demonstrated, although the opioid was not delivered locally at the site of inflammation but rather into the intraperitoneal cavity.

LA, local anaesthetic; NSAID, non-steroidal anti-inflammatory drug; VAS, visual analogue scale.

of administration have been reported. These include intraperitoneal, topical wound infiltration or corneal, intravesical or perineurial administration and around a tooth extraction. In all these diverse routes of administration, the opioids appear to relieve the hyperalgesia only if there is evidence of inflammation, if it is locally confined and if the opioids are delivered at the site of inflammation (Table 1.1).

Tolerance

The side effects of opioids commonly associated with systemic administration, such as tolerance and respiratory depression, could potentially be avoided through the use of peripherally administered opioids. Studies on the whole suggest a lack of tolerance with peripheral opioid analgesia (Ueda & Inoue 1999). Tolerance has been reported, but in models that did not employ inflammation (Kolesnikov & Pasternak 1999b) and have been shown to be reversed with concurrent use of an N-methyl-D-aspartate (NMDA) antagonist (Kolesnikov & Pasternak 1999a, 1999b). Others using bradykinin or thermal models of inflammation have not shown tolerance (Tokuyama *et al.* 1998; Nozaki-Taguchi & Yaksh 1999; Ueda & Inoue 1999). Clinically, no tolerance has been found to peripheral morphine analgesia, in the presence of endorphin-rich inflamed synovia (Stein *et al.* 1996). However, further evaluation is needed in this area.

Conclusion

This chapter has discussed the presence of opioid receptors and peptides in the peripheral nervous system in the normal and inflamed state. It would appear that, although in normal tissue there is little or no opioid peptide release, and few if any active and available receptors, the situation is dramatically different in inflammation. During inflammation, the opioid receptors on PSNs become active, upregulated and available. Opioid peptide-containing immune cells are specifically recruited and activated at the site of inflammation and release endogenous opioids. These then exert a neuroimmunomodulatory effect. Via the PSN, hyperalgesia is attenuated and the PSN release of tachykinins is reduced. The immune infiltrate is also modulated, although the evidence for a pro- or anti-inflammatory effect appears to be one of balance of the amount of opioid, and type and duration of the inflammation.

There are numerous animal models of inflammation demonstrating the analgesic efficacy or μ, δ and κ agonists, and a growing body of evidence for the therapeutic use of morphine applied locally to sites of painful inflammation. Although the local application of opioids induces an effective analgesia, the limitations will remain the need for repeated doses into the site of inflammation, which it is not always possible to achieve. The goal must remain the development and exploitation of systemically administered opioids with restricted access to the CNS or even site-directed trafficking of opioid-containing immune cells.

References

Aasbo V, Raeder JC, Grogaard B, Roise O (1996). No additional analgesic effect of intra articular morphine or bupivacaine compared with placebo after elective knee arthroscopy. *Acta Anaesthesiologica Scandinavica* **40**, 585–8

Andoh T, Itoh M, Kuraishi Y (1997). Nociceptin gene expression in rat dorsal root ganglia induced by peripheral inflammation. *NeuroReport* **8**, 2793–2796

Antonijevic I, Mousa SA, Schager M, Stein C (1995). Perineurial defect and peripheral opioid analgesia in inflammation. *Journal of Neuroscience* **15**, 165–172

Back IN & Finlay I (1995). Analgesic effect of topical opioids on painful skin ulcers [letter]. *Journal of Pain Symptom Management* **10**, 493

Barber A & Gottschlich R (1997). Central and peripheral nervous system: novel developments with selective non-peptide kappa opioid receptor agonist. *Medical Pediatric Review* **12**, 525–562

Binder W & Walker S (1998). The peripherally selective kappa-opioid agonist asimadoline attenuates adjuvant arthritis. *British Journal of Pharmacology* **124**, 647–654

Binder W, Carmody J, Walker J (2000). Effect of gender on anti-inflammatory and analgesic actions of two kappa-opioids. *Journal of Pharmacology and Experimental Therapeutics* **292**, 303–309

Bjornsson A, Gupta A, Vegfors M, Lennmarken C, Sjoberg F (1994). Intra-articular morphine for postoperative analgesia following knee arthroscopy. *Regional Anesthesia* **19**, 104–108

Bryant CJ, Harrison SD, Hopper C, Harris M (1999). Use of intra articular morphine for postoperative analgesia following TMJ arthroscopy. *British Journal of Oral and Maxillofacial Surgery* **37**, 391–396

Butcher EC & Picker LJ (1996). Lymphocyte homing homeostasis. *Science* **272**, 60–66

Cabot PJ, Carter L, Gaiddon C et al. (197). Immune cell derived beta endorphin. Production release and control of inflammatory pain in rats. *Journal of Clinical Investigation* **100**, 142–148

Carpenter KJ, Vithlani M, Dickenson AH (2000). Unaltered peripheral excitatory actions of nociceptin contrast with enhanced spinal inhibitory effects after carrageenan inflammation: an electrophysiological study in the rat. *Pain* **85**, 433–441

Coggeshall RE, Zhou S, Carlton SM (1997). Opioid receptors on peripheral sensory axons. *Brain Research* **764**, 126–132

Crain SM & Shen KF (1990). Opioids can evoke direct receptor-mediated excitatory effects on sensory neurons. *Trends in Pharmacological Science* **11**, 77–81

Dalsgaard J, Felsby S, Juelsgaard P, Froekjaer J (1994). Low dose intra articular morphine analgesia in day case knee arthroscopy: a randomized double blinded prospective study. *Pain* 56, 151–4

DeHaven Hudkins DL, Burgos LC, Cassel JA et al. (1999). Loperamide (ADL 2 1294) an opioid antihyperalgesic agent with peripheral selectivity. *Journal of Pharmacology and Experimental Therapeutics* **289**, 494–502

Earl JR, Claxson AW, Blake DR, Morris CJ (1994). Proinflammatory effects of morphine in the rat adjuvant arthritis model. *International Journal of Tissue Reaction* **16**, 163–170

Elhakim M, Nafie M, Eid A, Hassin M (1999). Combination of intra articular tenoxicam, lidocaine and pethidine for outpatient knee arthroscopy. *Acta Anaesthesiologica Scandinavica* **43**, 803–808

Frank GB & Sudha TS (1987). Effects of enkephalin applied intracellularly on action potential in vertebrate A and C nerve fibre axons. *Neuropharmacology* **26**, 61–66

Gold MS & Levine JD (1996). DAMGO inhibits prostaglandin E2-induced potentiation of a TTX-resistant Na current in rat sensory neurons in vitro. *Neuroscience Letters* **212**, 83–86

Graham NM, Shanahan MD, Barry P, Burgert S, Talkhani I (2000). Postoperative analgesia after arthroscopic knee surgery: a randomized prospective double blind study of intravenous regional analgesia versus intra articular analgesia. *Arthroscopy* **16**, 64–6

Green PG & Levine J (1992). Delta and kappa opioid agonists inhibit plasma extravasation induced by bradykinin in the knee joint of a rat. *Neuroscience* **49**, 129–133

Gupta A, Axelsson K, Allvin R *et al.* (1999). Postoperative pain following knee arthroscopy: the effects of intra articular ketorolac and/or morphine. *Regional Anesthesia and Pain Medicine* **24**, 225–230

Gurkan Y, Kilickan L, Buluc L, Muezzinoglu S, Toker K (1999). Effects of diclofenac and intra articular morphine/bupivacaine on postarthroscopic pain control. *Minerva Anesthesiologica* **65**, 741–745

Gyires K, Budavar I, Furst S, Molnar I (1985). Morphine inhibits the carrageenan induced oedema and the chemoluminescence of leucocytes stimulated by zymosan. *Journal of Pharmacy and Pharmacology* **37**, 100–104

Halford WP & Gebhart BM (1995). Functional role and sequence analysis of a lymphocyte orphan opioid receptor. *Journal of Neuroimmunology* **59**, 91–101

Hassan AHS, Przewlocki R, Herz A, Stein C (1992). Dynorphin a preferential ligand for kappa-opioid receptors is present in nerve fibers and immune cells within inflamed tissue. *Neuroscience Letters* **140**, 85–88

Hassan AHS, Ableitner A, Stein C, Herz A (1993). Inflammation of the rat paw enhances axonal transport of opioid receptors in the sciatic nerve and increases their density in the inflamed tissue. *Neuroscience* **55**, 185–195

Heijnen CJ, Kavelaars A, Ballieux RE (1991). Beta endorphin: cytokine and neuropeptide. *Immunological Reviews* **119**, 41–63

Helyes Z, Nemeth J, Pinter E, Szolcsanyi J (1997). Inhibition by nociceptin of neurogenic inflammation and the release of SP and CGRP from sensory nerve terminals. *British Journal of Pharmacology* **121**, 613–615

Henderson G & McKnight AT (1997). The orphan opioid receptor and its endogenous ligand nociceptin/orphanin FQ. *Trends in Pharmacological Science* **18**, 293–300

Hong Y & Abbott FV (1995). Peripheral opioid modulation of pain and inflammation in the formalin test. *Proceedings of the Royal Society of London Series B Biology* **277**, 1317–1327

Ingram SL & Williams JT (1994). Opioid inhibition on Ih via adenylyl cyclase. *Neuron* **13**, 179–186

Inoue M, Kobayashi M, Kozaki S, Zimmer A, Ueda H (1998). Nociceptin/orphanin FQ- induced nocieptive responses through substance P release form peripheral nerve ending in mice. *Proceedings of the National Academy of Sciences of the USA* **95**, 10949–10953

Ji RR, Zhang Q, Law PY, Low HH, Elde R, Hokfelt T (1995). Expression of mu delta and kappa opioid receptor like immunoreactivities in rat dorsal root ganglia after carrageenan induced inflammation. *Journal of Neuroscience* **15**, 8156–8166

Jin S, Lei L, Wang Y, Da D, Zhao Z (1999). Endomorphin-1 reduces carrageenan-induced fos expression in the rat spinal dorsal horn. *Neuropeptides* **33**, 281–284

Joshi GP, McCarroll SM, Brady OH, Hurson BJ, Walsh G (1993). Intra-articular morphine for pain relief after anterior cruciate ligament repair. *British Journal of Anaesthesia* **70**, 87–88

Kalso E, Tramer MR, Carroll D, McQuay HJ, Moore RA (1997). Pain relief from intra articular morphine after knee surgery: a qualitative systematic review. *Pain* **71**, 127–134

Khalil Z, Sanderson K, Modig M Nyberg F (1999). Modulation of peripheral inflammation by locally administered endomorphin-1. *Inflammation Research* **48**, 550–556

Khoury GF, Chen AC, Garland DE, Stein C (1992). Intraarticular morphine bupivacaine and morphine/bupivacaine for pain control after knee videoarthroscopy. *Anesthesiology* **77**, 263–266

Kinnman E, Nygards E-B, Hanson P (1997). Peripherally administered morphine attenuates capsaicin-induced mechanical hypersensitivity in humans. *Anesthesia and Analgesia* **84**, 822–826

Ko M-C, Butelman ER, Woods JH (1999). Activation of peripheral kappa opioid receptors inhibits capsaicin-induced thermal nociception in rhesus monkeys. *Journal of Pharmacology and Experimental Therapeutics* **289**, 378–385

Kolesnikov Y & Pasternak GW (1999a). Topical opioids in mice: analgesia and reversal of tolerance by a topical *N*-methyl-D-aspartate antagonist. *Journal of Pharmacology and Experimental Therapeutics* **290**, 247–252

Kolesnikov YA, Pasternak GW (1999b). Peripheral blockade of topical morphine tolerance by ketamine. *European Journal of Pharmacology* **374**, R1–R2

Kowalski J (1998). Immunologic action of [met5]enkephalin fragments. *European Journal of Pharmacology* **347**, 95–99

Krajnik M & Zylicz Z (1997). Topical morphine for cutaneous cancer pain [letter] [see comments]. *Palliative Medicine* **11**, 325

Krajnik M, Zylicz Z, Finlay I, Luczak J, van Sorge AA (1999). Potential uses of topical opioids in palliative care report of 6 cases. *Pain* **80**, 121–125

Laurent SC, Nolan P, Pozo JL, Jones CJ (1994). Addition of morphine to intra-articular bupivicaine does not improve analgesia after day-case arthroscopy. *British Journal of Anaesthesia* **72**, 170–173

Lawerence AJ, Joshi GP, Michalkiewicz A, Blunnie WP, Moriarty DC (1992). Evidence for analgesia mediated by peripheral opioid receptors in inflamed synovial tissue. *European Journal of Pharmacology* **43**, 351–355

Likar R, Mathiaschitz K, Burtscher, M Stettner H (1995). Randomised double blind comparative study of morphine and tramadol administered intra-articularly for postoperative analgesia following arthroscopic surgery. *Clinical Drug Investigation* **10**, 17–21

Likar R, Schafer M, Paulak F *et al.* (1997). intra-articular morphine analgesia in chronic pain patients with osteoarthritis. *Anesthesia and Analgesia* **84**, 1313–1317

Likar R, Sittl R, Gragger K *et al.* (1998). Peripheral morphine analgesia in dental surgery. *Pain* **76**, 145–50

Likar R, Kapral S, Steinkellner H, Stein C, Schafer M (1999). Dose dependency of intra articular morphine analgesia. *British Journal of Anaesthesia* **83**, 241–244

Machelska H, Binder W, Stein C (1999a). Opioid receptors in the periphery. In: Kalso E, McQuay H, Wiesenfeld-Hallin Z (eds) *Opioid Receptors in the Periphery*, vol. 14. Seattle: IASP Press pp 45–58

Machelska H, Pfluger M, Weber W *et al.* (1999b). Peripheral effects of the kappa opioid agonist EMD 61753 on pain and inflammation in rats and humans. *Journal of Pharmacology and Experimental Therapeutics* **290**, 354–61

Meunier J-C (1997). Nociceptin/orphanin FQ and the opioid receptor-like ORL1 receptor. *European Journal of Pharmacology* **340**, 1–15

Meunier J-C, Mollereau C, Toll L *et al*. (1995). Isolation and structure of the endogenous agonist of opioid receptor like ORL1 receptor [see comments]. *Nature* **377**, 532–535

Millan MJ & Colpaert FC (1991). Opioid systems in the response to inflammatory pain: sustained blockade suggests role of kappa- but not mu-opioid receptors in the modulation of nociception behaviour and pathology. *Neuroscience* **42**, 541–553

Moiniche S, Dahl JB, Kehlet H (1993). Peripheral antinociceptive effects of morphine after burn injury. *Acta Anaesthesiologica Scandinavica* 37 710–712

Mousa SA, Sachafer M, Mitchell WM, Hassan AHS, Stein C (1996). Local upregulation of corticotropin-releasing hormone and interleukin-1 receptors in rats with painful hindlimb. *European Journal of Pharmacology* **311**, 221–231

Niemi L (1994). Effects of intrathecal clonidine on duration of bupivacaine spinal anaesthesia haemodynamics and postoperative analgesia in patients undergoing knee arthroscopy. *Acta Anaesthesiologica Scandinavica* **38**, 724–728

Nothacker HP, Reinscheid RK, Mansour A *et al*. (1996). Primary structure and tissue distribution of the orphanin FQ precursor. *Proceedings of the National Academy of Sciences of the USA* **93**, 8677–8682

Nozaki-Taguchi N & Yaksh TL (1999). Characterization of the antihyperalgesic action of a novel peripheral mu-opioid receptor agonist-loperamide. *Anesthesiology* **90**, 225–234

Olsson Y (1990). Microenvironment of the peripheral nervous system under normal and pathological conditions. *Critical Review of Neurobiology* **5**, 265–311

Peluso J, LaForge KS, Matthes HW *et al*. (1998). Distribution of nociceptin/orphanin FQ receptor transcript in human central nervous system and immune cells. *Journal of Neuroimmunology* **81**, 184–192

Perrot S, Guilbaud G, Kayser V (1999). Effects of intraplantar morphine on paw oedema and pain related behaviour in a rat model of repeated acute inflammation. *Pain* **83**, 249–257

Peyman GA, Rahimy MH, Fernandes ML (1994). Effects of morphine on corneal sensitivity and epithelial wound healing: implications for topical ophthalmic analgesia. *British Journal of Ophthalmology* **78**, 138–141

Raja SN, Dickstein RE, Johnson CA (1992). Comparison of postoperative analgesic effects of intraarticular bupivacaine and morphine following arthroscopic knee surgery. *Anesthesiology* **77**, 1143–1147

Rodrigues AR & Duarte ID (2000). The peripheral and antinociceptive effect induced by morphine is associated with ATP-sensitive K(+) channels. *British Journal of Pharmacology* **129**, 110–114

Rorarius M, Suominen P, Baer G, Pajunen P, Tuimala R, Laippala P (1999). Peripherally administered sufentanil inhibits pain perception after postpartum tubal ligation. *Pain* **79**, 83–88

Rosseland LA, Stubhaug A, Skoglund A, Breivik H (1999). Intra articular morphine for pain relief after knee arthroscopy. *Acta Anaesthesiologica Scandinavica* **43**, 252–257

Russell NSW, Jamieson A, Calle A, Rance MJ (1985). Peripheral opioid effects upon neurogenic plasma extravasation and inflammation. *British Journal of Pharmacology* **84**, 788

Salzet M, Vieau D, Day R (2000). Crosstalk between nervous and immune systems through the animal kingdom: focus on opioids. *Trends in Neuroscience* **23**, 550–555

Samoriski GM & Gross RA (2000). Functional compartmentalization of opioid desensitization in primary sensory neurons. *Journal of Pharmacology and Experimental Therapeutics* **294**, 500–509

Sarne Y, Fields A, Gafni M (1996). Stimulatory effects of opioids on transmitter release and possible cellular mechanisms: overview and original results. *Neurochemistry Research* **21**, 1353–1361

Schafer MKH, Bette M, Romeo H, Schwaeble W, Weihe E (1994). Localisation of kappa-opioid receptor mRNA in neuronal subpopulations of rat sensory ganglia and spinal cord. *Neuroscience Letters* **167**, 137–140

Schafer M, Imai Y, Uhl GR, Stein C (1995). Inflammation enhances peripheral mu-opioid receptor mediated analgesia by not mu-opioid receptor transcription in the dorsal root ganglia. *European Journal of Pharmacology* **279**, 165–169

Schafer M, Mousa SA, Zhang Q, Carter L, Stein C (1996). Expression of corticotropin-releasing factor in inflamed tissue is required for intrinsic peripheral opioid analgesia. *Proceedings of the National Academy of Sciences of the USA* **93**, 6096–6100

Schafer M, Mousa SA, Stein C (1997). Corticotropin-releasing factor in antinociception and inflammation. *European Journal of Pharmacology* **323**, 1–10

Schinkel AH, Wagenaar E, Mol CAAM, van Deemter L (1996). P-glycoprotein in the blood-brain barrier of mice influences the brain penetration and pharmacological activity of many drugs. *Journal of Clinical Investigation* **97**, 2517–2524

Schulte Steinberg H, Weninger E, Jokisch *et al.* (1995) Intraperitoneal versus interpleural morphine or bupivacaine for pain after laparoscopic cholecystectomy. *Anesthesiology* **82**, 634–640

Selley DE, Breivogel CS, Childers SR (1993). Modification of G protein-coupled functions by low pH pretreatment of membranes from NG108–15 cells: increase in opioid agonist efficacy by decrease inactivation of G proteins. *Molecular Pharmacology* **44**, 731–741

Sharp B & Linner K (1993). What do we know about the expression of proopiomelancortin transcripts and related peptides in lymphoid tissue? *Endocrinology* **133**, 1921A–1921B

Sharp BM, Roy S, Bidlack JM (1998). Evidence for opioid receptors on cells involved in host defense and the immune system. *Journal of Neuroimmunology* **83**, 45–56

Sizemore RC, Dienglewicz RL, Pecunia E, Gottlieb AA (1991). Modulation of concanavalin A induced antigen nonspecific regulatory cell activity by leu enkephalin and related peptides. *Clinical Immunology and Immunopathology* **60**, 310–318

Stefano GB, Scharrer B, Smith EM *et al.* (1996). Opioid and opiate immunoregulatory processes. *Critical Review of Immunology* **16**, 109–144

Stein A, Yassouridis A, Szopko C, Helmke K, Stein C (1999). Intraarticular morphine versus dexamethasone in chronic arthritis. *Pain* **83**, 525–532

Stein C (1991). Peripheral analgesic actions of opioids. *Journal of Pain and Symptom Management* **6**, 119–124

Stein C (1993). Peripheral mechanisms of opioid analgesia. *Anesthesia and Analgesia* **76**, 182–191

Stein C (1995). Mechanisms of disease: the control of pain in peripheral tissue by opioids. *New England Journal of Medicine* **332**, 1685–1690

Stein C, Millan MJ, Shippenberg TS, Peter K, Herz A (1989). Peripheral opioid receptors mediating antinociception in inflammation: evidence for involvement of mu delta kappa receptors. *Journal of Pharmacology and Experimental Therapeutics* **248**, 1269–1275

Stein C, Hassan AHS, Przewlocki R, Gramsch C, Peter K, Herz A (1990). Opioids from immunocytes interact with receptors on sensory nerves to inhibit nociception in inflammation *Proceedings of the National Academy of Sciences of the USA* **87**, 5935–5939

Stein C, Comisel K, Haimerl E *et al.* (1991). Analgesic effect of intraarticular morphine after arthroscopic knee surgery [see comments]. *New England Journal of Medicine* **325**, 1123–1126

Stein C, Hassan AHS, Lehrberger K, Giefing J, Yassouridis A (1993). Local analgesic effect of endogenous opioid peptides. *The Lancet* **342**, 321–324

Stein C, Pfluger M, Yassouridis A (1996). No tolerance to peripheral morphine analgesia in presence of opioid expression in inflamed synovia. *Journal of Clinical Investigation* **98**, 793–799

Stein C, Schager M, Cabot PJ *et al.* (1997). Peripheral opioid analgesia. *Pain Reviews* **4**, 173–187

Taylor F & Dickenson AH (1998). Nociceptin/orphanin FQ. A new opioid a new analgesic? *NeuroReport* **9**, R56–R70

Tetzlaff JE, Dilger JA, Abate J, Parker RD (1999). Preoperative intra articular morphine and bupivacaine for pain control after outpatient arthroscopic anterior cruciate ligament reconstruction. *Regional Anesthesia and Pain Medicine* **24**, 220–224

Tokuyama S, Inoue M, Fughigami T, Ueda H (1998). Lack of tolerance in peripheral opioid analgesia in mice. *Life Science* **62**, 1677–1681

Twillman RK, Long TD, Cathers TA, Mueller DW (1999). Treatment of painful skin ulcers with topical opioids. *Journal of Pain and Symptom Management* **17**, 288–292

Ueda H & Inoue M (1999). Peripheral morphine analgesia resistant to tolerance in chronic morphine-treated mice. *Neuroscience Letters* **266**, 105–108

Varkel V, Volpin G, Ben David B *et al.* (1999). Intraarticular fentanyl compared with morphine for pain relief following arthroscopic knee surgery. *Canadian Journal of Anaesthesia* **46**, 867–871

Vaughan CW & Christie MJ (1996). Increase in the ORL1 receptor (opioid receptor like) ligand nociceptin of inwardly rectifying K conductance in dorsal raphe nucleus neurones. *British Journal of Pharmacology* **117**, 1609–1611

Vindrola O, Mayer AM, Citera G, Spitzer JA, Espinoza LR (1994). Prohormone convertases PC2 and PC3 in rat neutrophils and macrophages. Parallel changes with proenkephalin derived peptides induced by LPS in vivo. *Neuropeptides* **27**, 235–244

Walker JS, Chandler AK, Wilson JL, Binder W, Day RO (1996). Effect of mu-opioids morphine and buprenorphine on the development of adjuvant arthritis in rats. *Inflammation Research* **45**, 299–302

Weigent DA & Blalock JE (1997). Production of peptide hormones and neurotransmitters by the immune system. *Chemical Immunology* **69**, 1–30

Weihe E, Nohr D, Millan MJ (1988). Peptide neuroanatomy of adjuvant-induced arthritic inflammation in rat. *Agents and Actions* **25**, 255–259

Weisinger G (1995). The transcriptional regulation of the preproenkephalin gene. *Biochemical Journal* **307**, 617–629

Wenk HN & Honda CN (1999). Immunohistochemical localization of delta opioid receptors in peripheral tissues. *Journal of Comparative Neurology* **408**, 567–579

Wick MJ, Minnerath SR, Lin X, Elde R, Law P-Y, Loh HH (1994). Isolation of a novel cDNA encoding a putative membrane receptor with a high homology to the cloned mu delta and kappa opioid receptors. *(Brain Research) Molecular Brain Research* **27**, 37–44

Wick MJ, Minnerath SR, Ramakrishanan S, Loh HH (1995). Expression of alternate forms of brain opioid orphan receptor mRNA in activated human peripheral blood lymphocytes and lymphocytic lines. *(Brain Research) Molecular Brain Research* **32**, 342–347

Wilson JL, Nayanar V, Walker JS (1996). The site of anti-arthritic action of the kappa opioid U-50488H in adjuvant arthritis: importance of local administration. *British Journal of Pharmacology* **118**, 1754–1760

Wood A (1885). New method of treating neuralgia by the direct application of opiates to the painful points. *Edinburgh Medical and Surgical Journal* **82**, 265–281

Xie W, Samoriski GM, McLaughlin JP *et al.* (1999). Genetic alteration of phospholipase C beta 3 expression modulates behavioral and cellular responses to mu opioids. *Proceedings of the National Academy of Sciences of the USA* **96**, 10385–10390

Yoshino SI, Koiwa M, Shiga H, Nakamura H, Higaki M, Miyasaka N (1992). Detection of opioid peptides in synovial tissues of patients with rheumatoid arthritis. *Journal of Rheumatology* **19**, 660–661

Zhang Q, Schafer M, Elde R, Stein C (1998). Effects of neurotoxins and hindpaw inflammation on opioid receptor immunoreactivities in dorsal root ganglia. *Neuroscience* **85**, 281–291

Zhong F, Li XY, Yang SL, Stefano GB, Fimiani C, Bilfinger TV (1998). Methionine enkephalin stimulates interleukin 6 mRNA expression: human plasma levels in coronary artery bypass grafting. *International Journal of Cardiology* **64**(suppl), 1 S53–S59

Zhou L, Zhang Q, Stein C, Schafer M (1998). Contribution of opioid receptors on primary afferant versus sympathetic neurons to peripheral opioid analgesia. *Journal of Pharmacology and Experimental Therapeutics* **286**, 1000–1006

PART 2

Investigation and management of physical and non-physical pain

Chapter 2

The assessment and measurement of physical pain

Andrew Davies

Introduction

Pain is a subjective phenomenon (International Association for the Study of Pain or IASP 1986). Non-professional carers are relatively good at describing non-specific features of the pain (e.g. the presence of pain), but relatively poor at describing other features of the pain (e.g. the site of pain) (O'Brien & Francis 1988). Moreover, non-professional carers tend to overestimate the intensity of the patient's pain (Elliott *et al*. 1996). In contrast, professional carers tend to underestimate the intensity of the patient's pain (Grossman *et al*. 1991). Thus, ideally, the assessment and measurement of pain should be based on information provided by the patient, rather than on information provided by proxies.

Assessment of pain

Patients with cancer often have multiple pains, e.g. one study reported a median of 3 (range 1–11) different pains in a mixed group of palliative care patients (Twycross *et al*. 1996). Furthermore, patients with cancer often have multiple causes of pain. Indeed, the study by Twycross *et al*. (1996) reported that 46% of the pains were caused by a direct effect of the cancer, 29% by an indirect effect of cancer (i.e. secondary to debility), 5% by a direct/indirect effect of cancer treatment and 8% were unrelated to cancer. The cause of some of the pains in this study could not be determined.

The primary aim of assessment is to determine the aetiology of the pain, including pain's pathophysiology (e.g. nociceptive, neuropathic). Indeed, the aetiology of the pain determines its treatment. Thus, certain analgesics may not alleviate particular pains, e.g. opioid analgesics and the pain related to muscle spasm. Furthermore, certain analgesics may aggravate particular pains, e.g. opioid analgesics and the pain related to constipation.

The assessment of pain depends primarily on basic clinical skills, i.e. taking a history and performing an examination. It is important to take a general history, as well as a pain history. In particular, patients should be screened for psychological, spiritual and social factors that may be contributing to their experience of pain (the concept of 'total pain') (Twycross 1994). Similarly, it is important to perform a general examination, as well as an examination of the painful area. Investigations may also be of assistance in determining the aetiology of the pain.

The features of the pain that need to be determined include (Foley 1998):

- onset
- temporal pattern
- site
- radiation
- quality (i.e. character)
- intensity (i.e. severity)
- exacerbating factors
- relieving factors
- response to analgesics
- associated symptoms
- interference with activities of daily living.

A neurological examination of the painful area is mandatory (Portenoy 1997); the presence of neurological signs in the region of the pain suggests an underlying neuropathic component to the pain. It is usually possible to reproduce the patient's pain, and to identify the source of the patient's pain, by the use of 'provocative manoeuvres' such as palpation or passive movement (Hagen 1999).

The aetiology of pain often varies over time. Thus, the assessment of pain should be an ongoing process.

Measurement of pain

The primary aim of measurement is to determine the effectiveness of treatment for the pain. Various outcome measures have been used to assess treatment response, including: intensity of pain, distress of pain, pain relief, use of breakthrough medication, satisfaction with treatment, improvement in function and improvement in quality of life.

The different outcome measures relate to different aspects of the pain. Consequently, there is often a poor correlation between the results obtained with different outcome measures, e.g. in one study involving oncology patients, the percentage of patients who were 'inadequately treated' varied from 16% to 91%, depending on the specific outcome measure used (Table 2.1) (de Wit *et al*. 1999).

Table 2.1 Correlation between results obtained with different outcome measures (adapted from de Wit *et al.* 1999)

Outcome measure	Patients 'inadequately treated' (%)
Pain intensity (average)	60
Pain intensity (worst)	91
Pain relief	16
Patient satisfaction	32

All of the aforementioned outcome measures have limitations, e.g. pain relief is related to the change in pain intensity over a period of time – it is dependent on the patient's recollection of the baseline pain intensity. There is little consensus on the specific outcome measure that should be used to assess treatment response (de Wit *et al.* 1999).

Outcome measures are usually based on a verbal rating scale, a numerical rating scale or a visual analogue scale (Figure 2.1). Studies have shown a good correlation between the results obtained with these different scales (McQuay & Moore 1998); the relationship between the results obtained with these different scales is shown in Table 2.2. Outcome measures have also been based on pictorial scales, e.g. the 'faces' scales.

- Verbal rating scale, e.g. McGill Pain Questionnaire (Melzack 1975)

  No pain; mild; discomforting; distressing; horrible; excruciating

- Numerical rating scale, e.g. Brief Pain Inventory (Daut *et al.* 1983)

  A. Pain intensity

  0   1   2   3   4   5   6   7   8   9   10

  No   Pain as bad as
  pain   you can imagine

  B. Pain relief

  0%   10% 20% 30% 40%   50% 60% 70% 80% 90% 100%

  No   Complete
  relief   relief

- Visual analogue scale, e.g. Memorial Pain Assessment Card (Fishman *et al.* 1987)

  A. Pain intensity

  LEAST   _____   WORST
  possible pain   possible pain

  B. Pain relief

  NO   _____   COMPLETE
  relief of pain   relief of pain

Figure 2.1 Outcome measure scales.

Patients with advanced cancer often have difficulty in completing the outcome measures, e.g. in one study involving palliative care inpatients, 45% were unable to complete any of the relevant outcome measures (Shannon *et al.* 1995). Furthermore, of the remaining patients, 11% were unable to complete a categorical scale and 25% were unable to complete a visual analogue scale. The most common reason for being unable to complete the outcome measures was cognitive impairment.

Table 2.2 Relationship between results obtained with verbal rating scales, numerical rating scales and visual analogue scales

Verbal rating scale	Numerical rating scale[a] (0–10)	Visual analogue scale[b] (100 mm)
None	0	–
Mild	1–4	–
Moderate	5–6	> 30 mm (mean 49)
Severe	7–10	> 54 mm (mean 75)

[a]From Serlin *et al.* 1995
[b]From Collins *et al.* 1997

Studies suggest that the formal measurement of pain leads to the improved management of pain, e.g. in one study involving oncology outpatients, participants whose outcome measures were reveiwed were more likely to have had an improvement in their pain intensity at follow-up than those whose outcome measures were unavailable for review (Trowbridge *et al.* 1997).

The intensity of the pain often varies over time. Thus, the measurement of pain should also be an ongoing process.

Specific pain measurement tools

There are a variety of specific pain assessment/measurement tools, which have been validated in patients with cancer. These include the Brief Pain Inventory (long and short form) (Daut *et al.* 1983), the McGill Pain Questionnaire (long and short form) (Melzack 1975) and the Memorial Pain Assessment Card (Fishman *et al.* 1987).

The aforementioned specific pain measurement tools have similar limitations to the generic pain measurement tools. They are generally used in the research setting, rather than in the clinical setting.

Conclusion

The successful management of cancer pain depends on an adequate assessment of the pain, appropriate treatment and adequate assessment of the treatment (i.e. measurement of pain/pain relief).

Further research is required to determine the specific outcome measure that should be used to assess treatment response in patients with advanced cancer. In the meantime, patients in clinical trials should be monitored using one of the specific pain measurement tools, such as the Brief Pain Inventory. Other patients should be monitored using an appropriate outcome measure (see below).

The World Health Organization's guidelines on the management of cancer pain are based on the principles of: (1) by the mouth; (2) by the clock; (3) by the ladder; (4) for the individual; and (5) attention to detail (WHO 1996). The latter two principles are also applicable to the measurement of cancer pain, e.g. it would seem more appropriate to record the 'worst pain intensity' than the 'average pain intensity' in patients with paroxysmal/intermittent pain. Similarly, it would seem more appropriate to use a verbally administered numerical rating scale than a visual analogue scale in patients with visual impairment.

References

Collins SL, Moore A, McQuay HJ (1997). The visual analogue pain intensity scale: what is moderate pain in millimetres? *Pain* **72**, 95–97

Daut RL, Cleeland CS, Flanery RC (1983). Development of the Wisconsin Brief Pain Questionnaire to assess pain in cancer and other diseases. *Pain* **17**, 197–210

de Wit R, van Dam F, Abu-Saad HH *et al.* (1999). Empirical comparison of commonly used measures to evaluate pain treatment in cancer patients with chronic pain. *Journal of Clinical Oncology* **17**, 1280–1287

Elliott BA, Elliott TE, Murray DM, Braun BL, Johnson KM (1996). Patients and family members: the role of knowledge and attitudes in cancer pain. *Journal of Pain and Symptom Management* **12**, 209–220

Fishman B, Pasternak S, Wallenstein SL, Houde RW, Holland JC, Foley KM (1987). The Memorial Pain Assessment Card: a valid instrument for the evaluation of cancer pain. *Cancer* **60**, 1151–1158

Foley KM (1998). Pain assessment and cancer pain syndromes. In Doyle D, Hanks GWC, MacDonald N (eds) *Oxford Textbook of Palliative Medicine*, 2nd edn. Oxford: Oxford University Press, pp 310–331

Grossman SA, Sheidler VR, Swedeen K, Mucenski J, Piantadosi S (1991). Correlation of patient and caregiver ratings of cancer pain. *Journal of Pain and Symptom Management* **6**, 53–57

Hagen NA (1999). Reproducing a cancer patient's pain on physical examination: bedside provocative maneuvers. *Journal of Pain and Symptom Management* **18**, 406–411

International Association for the Study of Pain (1986). Classification of chronic pain. *Pain* **3**(suppl), 51–226

McQuay HJ, Moore RA (1998). *An Evidence-based Resource for Pain Relief*. Oxford: Oxford University Press

Melzack R (1975). The McGill Pain Questionnaire: major properties and scoring methods. *Pain* **1**, 277–299

O'Brien J & Francis A (1988). The use of next-of-kin to estimate pain in cancer patients. *Pain* **35**, 171–178

Portenoy RK (1997). The physical examination in cancer pain assessment. *Seminars in Oncology Nursing* **13**, 25–29

Serlin RC, Mendoza TR, Nakamura Y, Edwards KR, Cleeland CS (1995). When is cancer pain mild, moderate or severe? Grading pain severity by its interference with function. *Pain* **61**, 277–284

Shannon MM, Ryan MA, D'Agostino N, Brescia FJ (1995). Assessment of pain in advanced cancer patients. *Journal of Pain and Symptom Management* **10**, 274–278

Trowbridge R, Dugan W, Jay SJ *et al.* (1997). Determining the effectiveness of a clinical-practice intervention in improving the control of pain in outpatients with cancer. *Academic Medicine* **72**, 798–800

Twycross R (1994). *Pain Relief in Advanced Cancer*. Edinburgh: Churchill Livingstone

Twycross R, Harcourt J, Bergl S (1996). A survey of pain in patients with advanced cancer. *Journal of Pain and Symptom Management* **12**, 273–282

World Health Organization (1996). *Cancer Pain Relief*, 2nd edn. Geneva: WHO

Chapter 3

The nature of non-physical pain

Peter Speck

Introduction

Before examining the nature of non-physical pain it is important to understand what we mean by the word 'pain'. The International Association for the Study of Pain (IASP) has defined it as:

> An unpleasant sensory and emotional experience associated with actual or potential tissue damage or described in terms of such damage.

IASP (1979)

However, pain is a very subjective experience and it is important to recognise that the experience is what the person says it is and not what others think it ought to be. When assessing pain, therefore, it is important to ensure that you are listening to the patient and assessing what he or she is actually experiencing. Language becomes very important because the language we use to describe another person's experience can influence how we view and value that experience. In turn this will also influence how we act in response to it. Kearney (1996) describes the distinction between soul pain and depression as a result of an individual experiencing disconnectedness within him- or herself.

Similarly, it is helpful to distinguish between the words 'pain' and 'suffering'. Pain is often used to describe an experience that is more focused and specific. There is usually some understanding of the reason for the pain and some hope of relief. It is very much an individual experience. Suffering, by contrast, is usually associated with the loss of meaning, purpose or hope. The associations are often with decay and disintegration, and represent a global rather than an individual experience.

As an example of this, a mother was sitting by her young child who had a very distended abdomen because of a liver tumour. The child was in great discomfort and the mother said 'Can't you give him something for his pain?'. Several weeks later, when visiting the mother and child, it was clear that the child was pain free and had said he was quite comfortable. However, the mother said 'I can't bear to see him suffering'. The pain and discomfort were now a shared experience and something wider than the physical confines of the child's body.

There are frequently different perceptions of the experience of pain, depending on whether you are the patient, the carer or viewing it from the stance of the organisation. These different perceptions can affect the assessment, management and response to pain.

The patient and the family may be reluctant to report pain or to follow treatment recommendations. There may also be a fear of injections, addiction to medication or the side effects of treatment. For some patients, there may be a belief that pain is inevitable and must be accepted (Ward *et al.* 1993; Wallace *et al.* 1995). This may be reinforced by religious belief if pain is seen as deserved or meritorious in some way.

The physician may also be influential, as illustrated by Grossman *et al.* (1991) who showed the disparity between the rating of pain by the patient and that by the physician. Larue *et al.* (1995) reviewed the knowledge of pain control in a group of French oncologists and the way this influenced their morphine-prescribing habits. Rogers and Todd (2000) have also looked at the practice of consultant oncologists in an outpatient clinic. They found that, when patients were invited to talk about their symptoms, the physicians only listened to the 'right kind' of pain. If the 'right kind' of pain was *detected* the patient was recommended for cancer therapy; if the 'right kind' of pain was *suspected* the patient was sent for further clinical investigations. In other words, the oncologists were seeking to identify pain that would be amenable to a 'technical fix'.

Organisationally, there is evidence to show that the regular use of pain measurement tools can heighten the awareness of pain in all healthcare professionals. This can lead to a greater commitment to ensuring that it is treated adequately (International Association for the Study of Pain 1986).

What is non-physical pain?

In 1967, Cicely Saunders talked of 'total pain' and of the many factors that can feed into the pain experience, as well as the way in which aspects of the individual's life can be affected by pain. Figure 3.1 is based on Saunders' concept.

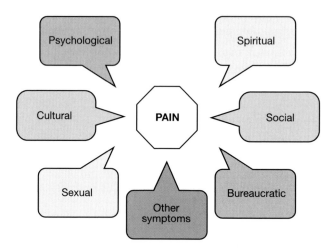

Figure 3.1 The concept of 'total' pain.

Dr Saunders' work highlighted the importance of careful assessment as to which factors are relevant to the patient and what might be appropriate responses to effect alleviation. Thus, some may require an intervention but there may be other factors with which the patient may feel he or she will live (or die) as an integral part of the person.

Other physical symptoms

Before you can begin to assess non-physical pain it is important to identify and, if possible, alleviate any physical symptoms that might contribute to the distress of the patient. These may include any one or more of the following – insomnia, exhaustion, persistent cough, repeat vomiting, hiccups, diarrhoea, dyspnoea, etc. – all of which may aggravate the perception of pain for the patient and the family.

Social factors

At a personal level, the individual may feel isolated or have unfinished business. There may also be distress at an interpersonal level because of tensions within the family or with others. Problems of self-care may become more significant because the patient has become more dependent, with the possible need for home care or a nursing home.

There may be financial or legal needs and the level of bureaucracy can lead to frustration, especially if life expectancy is short.

Psychological factors

The following are a number of psychological factors:

- Depression and anxiety, as distinct from transitory low mood, may be significant and correct differential diagnosis and treatment is important.
- Anger may sometimes be justified, and is not always grief or illness related.
- Grief for future loss of own life, loss of function, dignity, job, role or self-esteem, with a whole range of responses.
- Emotional exhaustion: this may result from fear of either further or future pain – the dying process. Previous experience of being with dying people can also affect this if the experience was not good.
- Loss of a coping strategy, 'fighting spirit' or faith, and a struggle to cope with diminishing emotional reserves can also be very distressing and lead to exhaustion in the person.

Sexual problems

These may be secondary to surgery, leading to loss of function or ability. The problems can be the result of the impact of disease or disfigurement or assumptions that sexual desire is not present or appropriate because of the illness. Sexual problems may also be the result of the attitudes of the partner, family or staff, indicating a taboo area that is not for discussion.

Hope

Hope is not necessarily related to the possibility of cure or long-term remission, but describes a quality of 'personhood' and being loved, accepted and valued.

Hope changes with time and is unique for each person because it links to re-defined goals and expectations.

Cultural factors

The patient or family may or may not express pain according to cultural norms within the family or society. Language can be a problem as can cultural attitudes towards morphine. It should be noted that stoicism may be the result of culture or religion.

Bates *et al.* (1993) looked at 372 patients with chronic pain, from six ethnic groups, who attended for treatment at a multidisciplinary pain management centre. They found that ethnocultural affiliation was important to pain perception and variation of response. The best predictors of pain intensity variation were ethnic group affiliation and locus of control style. They concluded that, although it was likely that intense pain affects attitudes and emotions, it is also very likely that attitudes and emotions influence reported perceptions of pain intensity. Greenwald (1991) studied 536 people recently treated for forms of cancer known to cause significant pain. The pain was assessed using standard, well-validated instruments, including graphic rating scales and the McGill Pain Questionnaire. Greenwald concluded that cultures associated with specific ethnic identities still condition individual expression of pain despite the high degrees of assimilation that have occurred among ethnic groups in the USA.

Spiritual, religious or philosophical beliefs

Distress is often the result of ill-formed beliefs or lack of meaning (in an existential sense) or unresolved questions, especially relating to the mystery of death.

Guilt and regrets about a past life can also cause distress. King *et al.* (1999) argued that re-structuring of the belief system in crisis can lead to vulnerability, although belief can also enable coping (Reed 1987; Kune *et al.* 1993; Koenig *et al.* 1998).

The *Oxford English Dictionary* defines spirituality as:

> A vital life principle which integrates other aspects of the person and is an essential ingredient in inter-personal relationships and bonding.

A serious and life-threatening illness, let alone the process of dying, has the power to threaten this integration and bonding. It is important to differentiate between the terms 'spiritual', 'religious', 'philosophical' and 'religiosity'. Most people who are religious are also spiritual. However, all those who are spiritual do not necessarily choose to express their spirituality in a religious format. Similarly, some people who are philosophical will wish to be described as spiritual whereas others do not. Some people will practise a religious ritual without any underpinning spirituality and, as such, would be best described as having religiosity. In assessing and offering spiritual care, one is, therefore, not necessarily offering it in a religious format or by a religious person.

How can we assess spiritual need and the presence, or absence, of spiritual pain or spiritual health?

The primary framework for assessing the many components leading to the experience of pain is within the clinical assessment:

- Believe the patient's complaint of pain
- Take a careful history
- Assess the character of each pain identified
- Clarify temporal aspects – acute, chronic, breakthrough, etc.
- List each pain according to the patient's priority
- Evaluate response to previous analgesia
- Evaluate psychological state and other influential factors
- Check previous alcohol/drug dependency
- Perform careful medical/neurological examination
- Provide continuity of care to reduce anxiety and increase compliance
- Then Review … Review … Review ….

(Adapted from Foley [1998])

Some of the key pain assessment tools include the various pain scales (visual and numeric), but also the variety of revised quality of life (QoL) scales and assessment tools.

A recent study undertaken in Cardiff by Pratheepawanit *et al.* (1999) compared two quality of life measures:

1. McGill QoL Questionnaire (MQoL): long, listing 16 items in 5 domains, including physical symptoms, physical well-being, psychological (existential and support).
2. Patient Evaluated Problem Scores (PEPS): much shorter than the MQoL.

There was a 60% preference for the MQoL because of its comprehensive natures and a 28% preference for the PEPS because of its simplicity.

Both instruments were found to be valid and reliable. The findings support the importance of an *existential* domain in assessing QoL in the palliative care population and to demonstrate its acceptability to patients. The Cardiff study recommends the regular use of such scales to prevent unsystematic clinical interviews.

Some information to enable an assessment of non-physical pain and its components has already been obtained during the course of the medical history taking, when information about the illness is obtained under the headings of past, present and future. Reviewing this information from a non-medical perspective can often yield valuable information for identifying wider issues (Speck 1998). The information that can be obtained is summarised below.

- Past (early symptoms): feelings of guilt/shame. Listen to the patient's story and knowledge and previous experience of cancer. This can raise issues of trust regarding present staff if previous experience was negative.
- Present (diagnosis): anger, suffering, coping strategies, spiritual health.
- Future (prognosis): hope – of cure? of treatment? For reconciliation, for a peaceful death?

If spiritual care is an integral component of *specialist* palliative care, it must be properly assessed. Timing is clearly important because it is often not possible to focus on wider issues until immediate concerns have been recognised, assessed and treated. This often includes the management of acute pain before other aspects of care can be assessed. Unfortunately, staff may too readily screen for religious need and assume that negative responses imply the absence of spiritual needs. As indicated earlier, people may have a spiritual belief system without expressing it in a religious way. King *et al.* (1999) indicate that 79% of patients interviewed during an acute, life-threatening illness demonstrated a spiritual and/or religious belief that was important to them and predictive of outcome from their disease.

However, many staff shy away from a more focused assessment of spiritual need because they are unsure what to explore once they move away from a more religious framework. The questions that one needs to explore must be more general and open-ended, so as not to lead the patient in a particular direction. Possible questions carers might ask include:

- Do you have a way of making sense of the things that happen to you?
- What sources of support or help do you look to when life is difficult? If this is religious what form does it take?
- Would you like to see someone who can help you talk or think through the impact of this illness or life event? (If the offered resource is a chaplain you may need to emphasise that the patient does not have to be religious to talk to them – the resource could instead be a clinical psychologist, nurse, doctor, social worker, etc.)

Conclusion

If we are to achieve better pain control for more patients then we will need:

- To ensure the optimal use of analgesics where chronic pain is the key issue.
- To explore other modes of treatment – which may include complementary approaches.
- To assess psychosocial/spiritual aspects effectively.

To meet the assessed needs, there needs to be a truly multidisciplinary and holistic approach. This is often maintained only if due attention is given to the dynamic processes within the staff group, otherwise they may ultimately be left bearing some of the patient's pain (Speck 1994).

References

Bates MS, Edwards WT, Anderson KO (1993). Ethnocultural influences on variation in chronic pain perception. *Pain* **52**, 101–112

Foley K (1998). Pain assessment and cancer pain syndromes. In Doyle D, Hanks GWC, Macdonald N (eds) *Oxford Textbook of Palliative Medicine*, 2nd edn. Oxford: Oxford University Press, pp 310–331

Greenwald HP (1991). Interethnic differences in pain perceptions. *Pain* **44**, 157–163

Grossman SA, Sheider VR, Swedeen K, Mucenski J, Piatadosi S (1991). Correlation of patient and caregiver ratings of cancer pain. *Journal of Pain and Symptom Management* **6**, 53–57

IASP Subcommittee on Taxonomy (1979). *Pain* **6**, 249–252

International Association for the Study of Pain (1986). Classification of chronic pain. *Pain* suppl 3, 51–226

Kearney M (1996). *Mortally Wounded – stories of soul pain, death and healing.* Marino: Dublin

King M, Speck P, Thomas A (1999). The effect of spiritual beliefs on outcome from illness. *Social Science & Medicine* **48**, 1291–1299

Kune GA, Kune S, Watson LF (1993). Perceived religiousness is protective for colorectal cancer. *Journal of the Royal Society of Medicine* **86**, 645–647

Koenig H, Pargament K, Nielsen J (1998). Religious coping and health status in medically ill hospitalised older adults. *Journal of Nervous and Mental Disease* **186**, 513–521

Larue F, Colleau SM, Fontaine A, Brasseur L (1995). Oncologists and primary care physicians' attitudes towards pain control and morphine prescribing in France. *Cancer* **76**, 2181–2185

Pratheepawanit N, Salek MS, Finlay IG (1999). The applicability of quality-of-life assessment in palliative care: comparing two quality-of-life measures. *Palliative Medicine* **13**, 325–334

Reed PG (1987). Spirituality and well-being in terminally ill hospitalised adults. *Research in Nursing and Health* **10**, 335–344

Rogers MS & Todd CJ (2000). The 'right kind' of pain: talking about symptoms in outpatient oncology consultations. *Palliative Medicine* **14**, 299–307

Saunders C (1967). *The Management of Terminal Illness.* London: Arnold

Speck P (1994). Working with dying people: on being good enough. In Obholtzer A & Zagier Roberts V (eds) *The Unconscious at Work.* London: Routledge, pp 94–100

Speck P (1998). Spiritual issues in palliative care. In Doyle D, Hanks GWC, Macdonald N (eds) *Oxford Textbook of Palliative Medicine*, 2nd edn. Oxford: Oxford University Press, pp 805–816

Wallace K, Reed B, Pasero C *et al.* (1995). Staff nurses' perceptions of barriers to effective pain management. *Journal of Pain and Symptom Management* **10**, 204–213

Ward SE, Goldberg N, Miller-McCauley V *et al.* (1993). Patient related barriers to management of cancer pain. *Pain* **52**, 319–324

PART 3

Evidence and opinion for opioid switching, co-analgesics and off-licence drugs

Scientific evidence and expert clinical opinion for the utility of opioid switching

Giovambattista Zeppetella and Claire Bates

Introduction

Pain in cancer patients is a complex problem with physical, social, psychological and spiritual dimensions. Physical pain is an important aspect of the total pain commonly experienced by cancer patients. Most patients with cancer pain will, however, respond to simple therapies. In 1986 the World Health Organization (WHO) published guidelines for cancer pain management based on the three-step analgesic ladder (WHO 1986). Since the WHO analgesic ladder was first proposed, there has been a wealth of clinical experience to support its use and studies have shown that adequate pain relief can be achieved in approximately 80% of patients (Hanks & Hawkins 2000).

The European Association for Palliative Care and the WHO recommend morphine as the opioid of choice for the management of moderate-to-severe pain (Expert Working Party of the European Association for Palliative Care 1996; WHO 1996). The dose of morphine should be titrated against the pain to achieve analgesia; a wide variation in mean daily dose has been reported (Boisvert & Cohen 1995). Morphine appears to have no clinically relevant ceiling effect to analgesia, but for some patients there may come a stage when further titration is made difficult because of unacceptable adverse effects. These adverse effects can include nausea, vomiting, sedation and hallucinations, which usually reduce within a few days, and constipation, which usually does not. It has been suggested that, for patients who appear unable to tolerate morphine, a switch to another opioid may be beneficial (Galer *et al.* 1992).

Opioids for moderate-to-severe pain

A number of alternatives to morphine are currently available and these include diamorphine, fentanyl, hydromorphone, oxycodone and methadone. The primary receptor binding for these drugs is shown in Table 4.1.

Morphine

Morphine, a potent μ agonist, was first isolated from the opium poppy in 1806 by the German pharmacist Frederich Sertürmer and its chemical structure determined in 1902. Morphine is now available in a wide range of formulations. After oral administration, the average bioavailability is 20–30%. Morphine is metabolised in

Table 4.1 Opioids and their primary receptor analgesic activity

Drug	Receptor type			
	μ	δ	κ	NMDA
Morphine	A	–	–	–
Diamorphine	A	–	–	–
Fentanyl	A	–	–	–
Hydromorphone	A	–	–	–
Methadone	A	–	A(?)	Ant
Oxycodone	A	A	–	–

NMDA, N-methyl-D-aspartate; A, agonist; Ant, antagonist.

the liver and the major metabolites are morphine-3-glucuronide (M3G) and morphine-6-glucuronide (M6G) (Yeh *et al.* 1977). M6G binds to opioid receptors and contributes to the analgesic effect of morphine, whereas M3G does not. In patients with normal renal function, morphine's plasma half-life is 2–3 hours whereas its duration of action is 4–6 hours. Caution is required in patients with renal impairment.

Diamorphine

Diamorphine is a semi-synthetic diacetyl derivative of morphine first synthesised in 1874. Its pharmacology is very similar to morphine but it is more soluble and lipophilic, which allows it to cross the blood–brain barrier more easily than morphine. Diamorphine has generally been considered to be devoid of analgesic activity itself (Inturrisi *et al.* 1984), although recent observations suggest the existence of a novel form of μ-receptor with which diamorphine, but not morphine, interacts (Rossi *et al.* 1996). Diamorphine is metabolised to 6-monoacetylmorphine, morphine and M6G. Clinically, the principal advantage of diamorphine over morphine is its greater solubility, which may be advantageous in subcutaneous administration. When administered by this route, diamorphine is approximately twice as potent as morphine (Kaiko *et al.* 1981).

Fentanyl

Fentanyl is a synthetic opioid agonist first introduced in 1960 as an anaesthetic. Fentanyl is primarily a μ agonist, with minor effects at κ- and δ-receptors. Fentanyl is approximately 80 times more potent than morphine and has a duration of action of 1–2 hours. It has a low molecular weight and high lipid solubility. There have been two recent formulations indicated for the management of cancer pain: Fentanyl TTS (Jeal & Benfield 1997), a transdermal preparation for the management of stable chronic pain, and oral transmucosal fentanyl citrate (Portenoy *et al.* 1999), developed for the management of breakthrough pain.

Hydromorphone

Hydromorphone is a semi-synthetic μ-opioid agonist first introduced in 1926 and recently available in the UK, although well established in the USA and Ireland. Hydromorphone has similar pharmacokinetic and pharmacodynamic properties to morphine but is more soluble, 5–10 times more potent (Lawlor *et al.* 1997) and has a half-life of 2–4 hours. Hydromorphone's bioavailability varies from 30% to 40% and the main metabolite is hydromorphone-3-glucuronide. Like diamorphine, it has a high solubility, which can make it particularly suitable for subcutaneous infusions.

Oxycodone

Oxycodone is a semi-synthetic opioid agonist first introduced in 1915. Its analgesic potency is approximately 25–50% greater than morphine (Heiskanen & Kalso 1997). In the USA oxycodone was originally combined with aspirin or acetominophen and therefore considered a WHO step 2 analgesic. Metabolised in the liver to noroxycodone, oxymorphone and various glucuronide conjugates, it has a bioavailability of 60–90% and a half-life of 2–4 hours. It has been suggested that oxycodone is less likely than morphine to cause hallucinations (Poyhia *et al.* 1993). Oxycodone has a lower affinity than morphine for the μ-receptor and recent studies indicate that oxycodone is a κ agonist (Ross & Smith 1997). It is preferred by some in the management of neuropathic pain (Watson & Babul 1998).

Methadone

A synthetic opioid developed in 1946 and included in the first draft of the WHO analgesic ladder, methadone's characteristics include lack of known active metabolites, generally long and unpredictable half-life, high lipid solubility, good absorption after oral and rectal administration and low cost. Its opioid activity includes μ and δ agonism, and there has been increasing interest more recently because of its putative *N*-methyl-D-aspartate (NMDA)-receptor antagonist effects (Ebert *et al.* 1995). Recent studies examining the equianalgesic dose of methadone to morphine suggests that methadone is more potent than originally described and that the ratio correlates with the total opioid dose before switching to methadone (Ripamonti *et al.* 1998). Methadone may be a useful alternative to morphine; however, its pharmacokinetics are complex and both dose and interval require careful titration for each patient.

Opioid receptors

The physical and chemical characteristics of morphine and related opioids led to the theory that they produce their effects by interacting with a specific receptor. Subsequently, in vivo studies demonstrated the spectrum of actions produced by different opioids, which, in turn, led to the suggestion that more than one type of opioid receptor was involved. It is now apparent that there are three well-defined opioid receptors: μ, δ and κ; genes encoding for these have been cloned. Three groups of endogenous opioids have also been discovered: β endorphins, enkephalins and dynorphins. Each group is derived from different polypeptide precursors and has different affinities for the distinct type of opioid receptors.

Opioid receptors have been classified by their selectivity in binding and in pharmacological assays and more recently through a series of selective antagonists. μ-Receptors were first defined by their high selectivity for morphine in pharmacological studies (Martin *et al.* 1976). They are thought to be responsible for most of the analgesic effects of opioids and for some major adverse effects (Table 4.2); most analgesics are μ-receptor agonists. δ-Receptors may be important in peripheral tissue but may also contribute to analgesia. κ-Receptors contribute to analgesia at a spinal level, and may produce sedation and dysphoria, but they produce fewer adverse effects. Some analgesics are κ-receptor selective. All three receptors are linked through G-proteins and after receptor activation a number of cellular mechanisms are produced, including inhibition of adenylyl cyclase, activation of potassium channels and inhibition of calcium channels. These effects reduce neuronal excitability and transmitter release. The overall effect is therefore inhibitory at the cellular level, although in some cases opioids can lead to an increase in neuronal activity, presumably by suppressing inhibitory interneurons.

Table 4.2 Functional effects associated with the main types of opioid receptors

Functional effect	μ	δ	κ
Analgesia			
– supraspinal	+++	–	–
– spinal	++	++	+
– peripheral	++	–	++
Pupillary constriction	++	–	+
Reduced gastrointestinal motility	++	++	+
Euphoria	+++	–	–
Dysphoria	–	–	+++
Sedation	++	–	++
Respiratory depression	+++	++	–

More recently an 'orphan' receptor has been identified and has been named ORL_1 (opioid receptor like). There is pharmacological evidence for subtypes of each receptor and other types of novel, less well-characterised opioid receptors ε, λ, ι, ζ have also been postulated. The σ-receptor was originally classified as an opioid receptor, although it now appears that these are not true opioid receptors but the site of action of certain psychomimetic drugs with which some opioids interact.

The discovery of multiple subclasses of opioid receptors in binding studies was soon followed by the demonstration of a number of discrete analgesic systems that were capable of independently relieving pain. Most clinically used analgesics relieve pain through more than one receptor mechanism. The receptor binding of a particular opioid is recognised as being important in drug efficacy. Opioids differ in the fraction of receptors that they need to occupy to achieve an equivalent effect; the greater the intrinsic activity of the drug the fewer the receptors that need to be occupied (Duttaroy & Yoburn 1995). Hence a drug with a higher receptor affinity such as fentanyl is capable of producing a maximal effect at lower receptor occupancy than a drug with a low receptor affinity such as morphine.

Clinical experience of opioid switching

The practice of changing to an alternative strong opioid when titration is made difficult as a result of adverse effects has come to be known as 'opioid rotation'. Alternative descriptions include opioid switching, sequential opioid trials and opioid substitution. The term 'opioid switching' was preferred at an expert meeting of the European Association for Palliative Care in 1998 and is therefore used here.

Clinical studies

There has been a growing body of literature in recent years describing the clinical use of opioid switching in case reports, prospective and retrospective studies. Different types of opioid switching have been described. These include:

- changing the opioid but not the route of administration
- changing the route of administration of the same opioid
- changing both the opioid and the route of administration.

Most of the literature reports on the use of methadone and hydromorphone as alternatives to morphine. Fewer studies describe switching to fentanyl and oxycodone and fewer still to sufentanil, dipipanone, levorphanol and ketobemidone (Galer *et al.* 1992; Faull *et al.* 1994; Sjogren *et al.* 1994; Hagen & Swanson 1997). The variation in the availability of different opioids between countries is obviously reflected in the choice of opioid when switching.

Reports involving methadone describe its successful use in patients with both nociceptive and neuropathic pain poorly responsive to high-dose morphine and hydromorphone, or in patients developing unacceptable toxicity with the original opioid. Some describe the gradual reduction of the initial opioid with concurrent titration of the methadone (Vigano *et al.* 1996). Others perform a straightforward switch replacing morphine/ hydromorphone with methadone at variable starting doses (Galer *et al.* 1992; Crews *et al.* 1993; Leng & Finnegan 1994; Thomas & Bruera 1995; Fitzgibbon & Ready 1997; Daeninck & Bruera 1999; Scholes *et al.*

1999). One report demonstrates the efficacy of the true 'rotation' of opioid: the sequential repeated use of hydromorphone and methadone (Vigano *et al*. 1996). Most of the studies report administering the methadone orally, although rectal (Bruera *et al*. 1995, 1996; Lawlor *et al*. 1998) and parenteral (Crews *et al*. 1993; Fitzgibbon & Ready 1997) routes are also documented.

Reports involving hydromorphone involve oral and parenteral administration and include successful switches from morphine to hydromorphone (Foley 1985; Galer *et al*. 1992; Bruera *et al*. 1996), methadone to hydromorphone (Vigano *et al*. 1996) and hydromorphone to morphine (Bruera & Schoeller 1992; Macdonald *et al*. 1993; de Stoutz *et al*. 1995; Bruera *et al*. 1996). These encompass broad dose ranges of hydromorphone, e.g. 6 mg to 2,076 mg of subcutaneous hydromorphone daily (Bruera *et al*. 1996).

Fentanyl as a transdermal patch affords effective analgesia in many patients with stable analgesic requirements. Experience suggests that switching patients to transdermal fentanyl is a clinical therapeutic decision taken fairly frequently in many palliative care units. Reviewing the literature it seems that fentanyl causes less constipation and drowsiness than morphine (TTS Fentanyl Multicentre Study Group 1994; Ahmedzai & Brooks 1997). It may also be less emetogenic, although this is less consistently documented (TTS Fentanyl Multicentre Study Group 1994; Paix *et al*. 1995). Successful opioid switching to fentanyl has been reported to relieve opioid toxicity and/or improve pain control (De Laat *et al*. 1997; Ellershaw *et al*. 1998; P McNamara unpublished observations). Although the transdermal preparation is the more commonly prescribed form, studies also describe successful switching to subcutaneous fentanyl infusions, resulting in stable or improved pain control and decreased toxicity (Paix *et al*. 1995; Watanabe *et al*. 1998). The fact that fentanyl is almost entirely eliminated by conversion in the liver to inactive metabolites also makes it a useful option for renally impaired patients who are vulnerable to the neurotoxicity caused by morphine's metabolites (Kirkham & Pugh 1995; Mercadente *et al*. 1997a). The available published data include a study that showed that an individual patient's responses to different opioids can be highly variable, predominantly in terms of the side-effect profiles experienced (Woodhouse *et al*. 1999).

Two studies have reported successful switching from morphine or hydromorphone to oxycodone (Maddocks *et al*. 1996; Gagnon *et al*. 1999). In both cases, oxycodone was administered parenterally and benefits were noted in toxicity reduction after the switch (see below).

When faced with opioid toxicity, some clinicians change the drug and others change the route of administration whereas others still change both the drug and the route (Cherny *et al*. 1995). Kalso *et al*. (1996) conducted a randomised, double-masked, cross-over study to compare the effectiveness and acceptability of epidural and subcutaneous morphine administration, and showed that both treatments provided better pain relief with less adverse effects compared with oral morphine.

Switching from morphine to Fentanyl TTS has also shown improvement in adverse effects (TTS Fentanyl Multicentre Study Group 1994). There is little evidence involving switching to diamorphine, probably because of its limited use outside the UK.

Opioid toxicity

The literature suggests that there are some notable differences in the frequency with which different centres use opioid switching to manage clinical situations where the adverse opioid effects become intolerable. One paper described the use of opioid switching (mainly for toxicity reduction) in 40% of patients admitted to a specialist palliative care unit (de Stoutz *et al.* 1995). Other authors suggest that the incidence of intolerable adverse opioid effects in patients receiving regular morphine is only 2–3% (Hawley *et al.* 1998), and that in these patients resolution of the adverse effects, while maintaining adequate analgesia, could be achieved by reducing the dose of the opioid so that opioid switching is necessary in relatively few cases.

Much has been written about the adverse effects of opioids on the central nervous system. Up to 25% of patients treated with morphine may experience acute delirium (Maddocks *et al.* 1996). Indeed, opioids can cause or aggravate delirium. Cognitive failure is the most characteristic feature, manifesting as decreased attention to outside stimuli, disorganised thinking, memory impairment, and disorientation in time, place and person. Two studies demonstrate improvement in cognitive state/delirium with switching to oxycodone (Maddocks *et al.* 1996; Gagnon *et al.* 1999). De Stoutz *et al.* (1995) record improvement in 66% of patients with cognitive failure and 66% of patients with hallucinations, using morphine, methadone and hydromorphone as alternative drugs. They also document 100% improvement in myoclonus with opioid switching. It is interesting that renal failure was associated with toxicity in only 20% of patients at the time of switching the opioid.

'Organic hallucinosis' is a term used to describe hallucinations in the presence of clear consciousness and intact intellectual functioning. There are case reports of opioid switching improving this specific opioid-induced neurological adverse effect, although the addition of an antipsychotic in each case may have clouded the picture (Bruera & Schoeller 1992).

Although the focus has been on the use of opioid switching for reduction of neurotoxic effects, there is evidence that opioid gastrointestinal adverse effects (constipation, nausea and vomiting) are also improved with switches to oxycodone or fentanyl (Maddocks *et al.* 1996; Ellershaw *et al.* 1998; Daeninck & Bruera 1999).

Dose equivalents

As the volume of literature on opioid switching has increased, it has emerged that clinical observations of equianalgesic doses often differ from doses predicted by previously calculated dose ratios. Most of the evidence used to calculate dose equivalence involved relatively low-dose studies. This evidence may not hold true in all patients, especially those on higher opioid doses. Macdonald *et al.* (1993) reported three cases where patients experiencing severe adverse effects with high-dose hydromorphone were switched successfully to morphine at 20–25% of the usually accepted equivalent dose, confirming the need for caution in the use of equianalgesic tables where high doses of opioids are concerned. There is some evidence that the initial dose of the first opioid influences the switch dose; Bruera *et al.* (1996) found that the hydromorphone : methadone ratio changed according to the total dose of hydromorphone that the patient was receiving before the switch (correlation coefficient 0.41, $p < 0.001$).

This phenomenon is perhaps best demonstrated in switches involving methadone. In the past, methadone was considered equianalgesic to morphine. In comparing methadone, hydromorphone and morphine, Bruera *et al.* (1996) found that dose ratios between morphine and hydromorphone, and vice versa, were 5.33 and 0.28, respectively – similar to expected results. However, the hydromorphone : methadone ratio was found to be 5–10 times higher than expected. Other studies have shown that large reductions in opioid dose can occur when switching to methadone, suggesting that methadone is much more potent than previously thought (de Stoutz *et al.* 1995; Fitzgibbon & Ready 1997). Furthermore, the equianalgesic dose may vary depending on the previous dose of morphine (Ripamonti *et al.* 1998) and on which opioid is given first (Lawlor *et al.* 1997).

The study of Bruera *et al.* (1996) comparing equianalgesic doses also observed a wide range in dose ratio for each of the three drugs, confirming that patients should be individually titrated to their optimal opioid dose. Other authors make the point that the interindividual variations in analgesic effect and side-effect profiles make extrapolation of single or limited case studies to larger populations extremely difficult (Vigano *et al.* 1996).

The equianalgesic dose of the opioid chosen may therefore be uncertain for various reasons. It will depend not only on the opioids being used, but also on the individual patient, the degree of cross-tolerance and the nature of the pain (Fallon 1997). The patient in the higher-dose range is potentially at greater risk of the equianalgesic dose being several-fold different than expected.

Other views

Not everyone supports the routine use of opioid switching. Fallon (1997) stressed the importance of thorough clinical assessment (including correction of abnormal biochemistry), use of appropriate co-analgesics, avoidance of sustained-release opioid preparations and the use of haloperidol to counteract the altered sensorium secondary to opioid toxicity. She argued that inappropriate opioid prescribing could shift a patient to the less responsive end of the continuum of opioid responsiveness (Fallon 1997). Others have endorsed this approach; Hawley *et al.* (1998) performed a retrospective study examining the incidence of opioid-induced confusion in hospital palliative care patients. Of the 57 patients found to be confused, opioids were thought to be 'a major causative factor' in 13. In 11 of these patients, the confusion resolved with a reduction in the opioid dose, the remaining 2 patients dying before any therapeutic changes could be implemented. These data supported the authors' opinion that opioid switching is necessary in less than 2–3% of patients taking strong opioids. A prospective study is currently under way (GW Hanks, personal communication).

Twycross (1998) has suggested that switching opioids might be appropriate in only two 'distinct syndromes'. First, opioid-induced cognitive failure (e.g. agitated delirium ± hallucinations ± sedation) at typical doses of the opioid in question, usually morphine or hydromorphone (Maddocks *et al.* 1996), which may reflect an idiosyncratic hypersensitivity to morphine. Second, opioid-induced hyperexcitability (multifocal myoclonus, jerking lower limbs, abdominal muscle spasms, hyperalgesia or whole-body allodynia, delirium and agitation), which is generally seen only with very high parenteral or spinal doses (De Conno *et al.* 1991; Sjogren *et al.* 1994; Hagen & Swanson 1997).

At present, the literature includes description of practice that differs substantially from one centre to another and data for randomised controlled trials are lacking. Interpreting the findings of the studies must take into account the different patient populations studied, the different patterns of analgesic use and the complexity of the underlying pain syndromes involved.

Rationale for opioid switching

A number of mechanisms have been proposed to account for observed improvement after opioid switching. These mechanisms are supported by animal and human studies and can be divided into genetic factors, pain mechanisms, tolerance and the role of opioid metabolites.

Genetic factors

Patients vary enormously in their analgesic needs. This variability is oftentimes ascribed to cultural and psychological difference, but evidence for a genetic component has been mounting. Genetic differences in opioid sensitivity in animals can be very dramatic (Baran *et al.* 1975; Pick *et al.* 1991), e.g. some mouse strains are deficient in their expression of μ receptors and are correspondingly insensitive to the analgesic effects of morphine (Vaught *et al.* 1988). Furthermore, the sensitivity of the various opioid subtypes appears to be under independent control (Moskowitz & Goodman 1985).

In humans, genetic differences have been demonstrated, e.g. the *O*-demethylation of codeine to morphine (Chen *et al.* 1988; Yue *et al.* 1989). Genetic differences in receptor affinities and densities, or efficiency of secondary messenger systems, could also lead to a variation in opioid responsiveness, although these have yet to be studied in humans. The importance of cultural, emotional and social factors makes studies of genetic sensitivity of patient groups difficult. However, the potential of genetic variability should reinforce the need to individualise the treatment of patients and their pain.

Pain mechanism

The variation in response to different opioids may be influenced by the pain mechanism. Animal studies have demonstrated that this mechanism may be related to the opioid receptor subtype (Schmauss & Yaksh 1984). Thus, the analgesic efficacy of a particular opioid agonist could vary depending on the nature of the pain. Patients may respond differently to alternative opioids, depending on the drug's affinity or efficacy at the receptor subtype, which is most important in mediating analgesia for a specific type of pain.

It is generally accepted that not all pain types respond equally to opioids. It has been suggested that there is a continuum of opioid responsiveness and that neuropathic pain, which is itself a heterogeneous pain state (Sindrup & Jensen 1999), is at the least sensitive end of the spectrum (Wall 1990). Twycross (1998) has defined the issue of variable analgesic response to different opioids by distinguishing between 'narrow-spectrum' opioids with predominantly μ activity (morphine, hydromorphone, oxycodone and fentanyl) and 'broad-spectrum' opioids with both μ- and δ-agonist activity (methadone and levorphanol). The proposed NMDA antagonist activity of methadone could imply greater efficacy in neuropathic pain (Makin *et al.* 1998).

The opioid responsiveness of neuropathic pain may be difficult to predict. Galer *et al.* (1992) reported two cases with typical neuropathic pain, which did not respond to morphine but were successfully treated with an alternative opioid. If morphine had been the only opioid administered, their unsuccessful outcome could have been interpreted as opioid unresponsiveness. Further evidence for opioid responsiveness comes from a survey of 593 cancer patients referred to a pain service and treated using the WHO ladder. A substantial number of neuropathic pains were successfully managed with analgesics and without the use of adjuvants (Grond *et al.* 1999).

Tolerance

A decreased responsiveness to the pharmacological effects of a drug resulting from a previous exposure is known as tolerance. In this case, tolerance refers to the need to increase the dose of analgesic in order to obtain the same effect. The need for escalating doses is a complex phenomenon and has been demonstrated experimentally in both animals and humans. Animal studies have demonstrated that tolerance occurs with all opioids regardless of the receptor class involved. Tolerance develops independently for each receptor system (Paul *et al.* 1990), at varying rates and to varying extents across receptor subtypes (Ling *et al.* 1989). It also varies across receptor types for different opioids (Sosnowski & Yaksh 1990), irrespective of the opioid's potency (Kissin *et al.* 1991). This may occur as a result of different affinities for receptor subtypes (Moulin *et al.* 1988). The lack of so-called cross-tolerance among various receptor classes provides further evidence for distinct analgesic systems and may help explain some clinically relevant issues.

True pharmacological tolerance to the analgesic effects of opioids is not a common clinical problem. Although there is some evidence to suggest that tolerance to analgesia effects can occur (Houde *et al.* 1966), most patients reach a dose that remains constant for prolonged periods (Schug *et al.* 1992; Collin *et al.* 1993; Mercadente *et al.* 1997b). The need for escalating doses usually results from disease progression rather than true analgesic tolerance. In fact, multiple factors, including pain intensity, type of pain, pharmacokinetic and genetic factors, are likely to play a role in dose escalation. Clinically, tolerance to the non-analgesic effects of opioid appears to occur commonly, albeit at varying rates and for different effects. Such tolerance is not a clinical problem but is in fact desirable because it allows effective titration to proceed. A patient could experience a favourable change if there is less cross-tolerance at the receptors mediating analgesia than those mediating adverse effects. It is apparent that various types of pain are more likely to activate certain opioid receptor mechanisms and therefore the degree to which tolerance develops may also, in part, be related to the type of pain stimulus. The mechanism of opioid tolerance remains unclear. Although some evidence from tissue culture studies reveals decreased secondary messenger systems, other studies have implicated the activation of antagonistic neuronal systems. The NMDA receptor antagonist MK801 has been shown to prevent tolerance to morphine (Trujillo & Akil 1991).

Opioid metabolites

Opioid metabolites may play a role in the observations seen when switching opioids. Differences in absorption, metabolism and excretion of morphine, for example, may account for part of the variability of the analgesic effect and adverse effects in cancer patients, e.g. morphine is principally metabolised to M3G and M6G. Some authors have suggested that the clinical analgesic effects are determined by the ratio M3G : M6G (Bowsher 1993; Morley *et al.* 1993), but this is not universally accepted. M6G is generally accepted to be a more potent analgesic than morphine itself (Paul *et al.* 1989; Hanna *et al.* 1990), whereas M3G, the main glucuronide, shows no analgesic activity. It has been suggested that M3G could combine with morphine and M6G and contribute to the morphine-induced hyperalgesia, allodynia and myoclonus described in cancer patients receiving high doses of morphine (Sjogren *et al.* 1993). Others have suggested that M3G activates the NMDA receptor complex, but binding studies show that M3G has a low affinity for known NMDA-binding sites (Bartlett *et al.* 1994). In addition to the opioid activity, high doses of morphine and/or its metabolites have an antiglycinergic effect in dorsal horn neurons, causing reduction in postsynaptic inhibition that results in hyperalgesia and myoclonus (Beyer *et al.* 1985).

Impaired liver function does not usually lead to significant changes in the actions of morphine, whereas renal failure may lead to accumulation of both M3G and M6G (Osborne *et al.* 1986). Age, sex and concomitant drugs may also affect the level of metabolites (McQuay *et al.* 1990). Adverse effects have been attributed to the levels of these metabolites in morphine and in other drugs such as hydromorphone (Macdonald *et al.* 1993). Switching to an alternative opioid could allow the offending metabolites to be excreted, although subsequent opioid metabolites could also accumulate. Some have argued that by continually switching, or rotating, opioids the level of metabolite levels is kept low. It would also be possible to rotate to the original opioid once its metabolites had been eliminated. Theoretically, opioids without known active metabolites may be associated with fewer side effects.

Conclusion

Most patients with cancer will have their pain well controlled using the WHO analgesic ladder. When pain control is compromised by adverse effects, a thorough clinical reassessment is necessary to determine the possible causes. A number of options then follow, including a review of the opioid regimen (dose, preparation and use of rescue medication), management of the adverse effects, and the use of pharmacological and non-pharmacological adjuvant therapies.

In some patients, switching opioids may be useful; the frequency with which this is practised will vary from one unit to another. At present, there is no evidence to suggest which opioid to switch to, and the decision is likely to be made on the grounds of availability, familiarity, convenience, patient preference and cost. Care is required when choosing the dose of an alternative opioid because it appears that this can vary widely and equianalgesic tables should serve only as a guide. Based on the clinical experience to date, it is not possible to state whether switching opioid is better than switching route of administration or whether there is any advantage of rotation over switching. The place of prophylactic rotation also needs clarification.

There has been some controversy surrounding the place of opioid switching in modern palliative medicine. Evidently the picture is still somewhat confused. This may reflect different units' contrasting patient populations and the different use of analgesics and adjuvant therapies. These factors should be taken into account when comparing available data and when planning future studies. Some answers will come through a better understanding of genetics and neuropharmacology. In the meantime, opioid responsiveness should be considered a dynamic event, which can change over time. Therefore, when faced with a patient with troublesome opioid-related adverse effects, regular reassessment of the clinical situation is always necessary.

References

Ahmedzai S & Brooks D (1997). Transdermal fentanyl versus sustained release oral morphine in cancer pain: preference, efficacy and quality of life. *Journal of Pain and Symptom Management* **13**, 254–261

Baran A, Shuster L, Eleftheriou BE, Bailey DW (1975). Opiate receptors in mice: genetic differences. *Life Sciences* **17**, 633–640

Bartlett SE, Cramond T, Smith MT (1994). The excitatory effects of morphine-3-glucuronide are attenuated by LY274614, a competitive NMDA receptor antagonist, and by midazolam, an antagonist at the benzodiazepine site on the $GABA_A$ receptor complex. *Life Sciences* **54**, 687–694

Beyer C, Roberts LA, Komisaruk BR (1985). Hyperalgesia induced by altered glycinergic activity at the spinal cord. *Life Sciences* **37**, 875–882

Boisvert M & Cohen SR (1995). Opioid use in advanced malignant disease: why do different centres use vastly different doses? A plea for standardized reporting. *Journal of Pain and Symptom Management* **10**, 632–638

Bowsher D (1993). Paradoxical pain. *British Medical Journal* **306**, 473–474

Bruera E & Schoeller T (1992). Organic hallucinosis in patients receiving high doses of opiates for cancer pain. *Pain* **48**, 397–399

Bruera E, Watanabe S, Faisinger RL, Spachynski K, Suarez-Almazor M, Inturrisi C (1995). Custom made capsules and suppositories of methadone for patients on high-dose opioids for cancer pain. *Pain* **62**, 141–146

Bruera E, Pereira J, Watanabe S, Belzile M, Kuehn N, Hanson J (1996). Opioid rotation in patients with cancer pain. A retrospective comparison of dose ratios between methadone, hydromorphone and morphine. *Cancer* **78**, 852–857

Cherny NJ, Chang V, Frager G *et al.* (1995). Opioid pharmacotherapy in the management of cancer pain: a survey of strategies used by pain physicians for the selection of analgesic drugs and routes of administration. *Cancer* **76**, 1283–1293

Chen ZR, Somogyi AA, Bochner F (1988). Polymorphic *O*-demethylation of codeine. *The Lancet* **ii**, 914–915

Collin E, Poulain P, Gauvain-Piquard A, Petit G, Pichard-Leandri E (1993). Is disease progression the major factor in morphine 'tolerance' in cancer pain treatment? *Pain* **55**, 319–326.

Crews JC, Sweeny NJ, Denson DD (1993). Clinical efficacy of methadone in patients refractory to other mu-opioid receptor agonist analgesics for management of terminal cancer pain. Case presentations and discussion of incomplete cross-tolerance among opioid agonist analgesics. *Cancer* **72**, 2266–2272

Daeninck PJ & Bruera E (1999). Reduction in constipation and laxative requirements following opioid rotation to methadone: a report of four cases. *Journal of Pain and Symptom Management* **18**, 303–309

De Conno F, Caraceni A, Martini C, Spoldi E, Salvetti M, Ventafridda V (1991). Hyperalgesia and myoclonus with intrathecal infusion of high-dose morphine. *Pain* **47**, 337–339

De Laat M, Deene P, Devulder J, Rolly G (1997). Advantages and limitations of transdermal fentanyl for pain management in terminal cancer patients (abstract). Fifth Congress of the European Association for Palliative Care

de Stoutz ND, Bruera E, Suarez-Almazor M (1995). Opioid rotation for toxicity reduction in terminal cancer patients. *Journal of Pain and Symptom Management* **10**, 378–384

Duttaroy A & Yoburn BC (1995). The effect of intrinsic efficacy on opioid tolerance. *Anesthesiology* **82**, 1226–1236

Ebert B, Andersen S, Krogsgaard-Larsen P (1995). Ketobemidone, methadone and pethidine are non-competitive N-methyl-D-aspartate (NMDA) antagonists in the rat cortex and spinal cord. *Neuroscience Letters* **187**, 165–168

Ellershaw JE, Smith JC, O'Donnell V, Murphy D, Halliwell B (1998). Opioid substitution with transdermal fentanyl (abstract). *Palliative Medicine* **12**, 489

Expert Working Party of the European Association for Palliative Care (1996). Morphine in cancer pain: modes of administration. *British Medical Journal* **312**, 823–826

Fallon M (1997). Opioid Rotation: does it have a role? *Palliative Medicine* **11**, 177–178

Faull C, McKechnie E, Riley J, Ahmedzai S (1994). Experience with dipipanone elixir in the management of cancer related pain – case study. *Palliative Medicine* **8**, 63–65

Fitzgibbon DR & Ready LB (1997). Intravenous high dose methadone administered by patient controlled analgesia and continuous infusion for the treatment of cancer pain refractory to high-dose morphine. *Pain* **73**, 259–261

Foley KM (1985). The treatment of cancer pain. *New England Journal of Medicine* **313**, 84–95

Gagnon B, Bielech M, Watanabe S, Walker P, Hanson J, Bruera E (1999). The use of intermittent subcutaneous injections of oxycodone for opioid rotation in patients with cancer pain. *Supportive Care in Cancer* **7**, 265–270

Galer BS, Coyle N, Pasternak GW, Portenoy RK (1992). Individual variability in the response to different opioids: report of five cases. *Pain* **49**, 87–91

Grond S, Radbruch L, Meuser T, Sabatowski R, Loick G, Lehmann KA (1999). Assessment and treatment of neuropathic cancer pain following WHO guidelines. *Pain* **79**, 15–20

Hagen N & Swanson R (1997). Strychnine-like multifocal myoclonus and seizures in extremely high-dose opioid administration: treatment strategies. *Journal of Pain and Symptom Management* **14**, 51–58

Hanks GW & Hawkins C (2000). Agreeing a gold standard in the management of cancer pain: the role of opioids. In Hillier R, Finlay I, Welsh J, Miles A (eds) *The Effective Management of Cancer Pain*. London: Aesculapius Medical Press, pp 57–77

Hanna MH, Peat SJ, Woodham M, Knibb A, Fung C (1990). Analgesic efficacy and CSF pharmacokinetics of intrathecal morphine-6-glucuronide: comparison with morphine. *British Journal of Anaesthesia* **64**, 547–550

Hawley P, Forbes K, Hanks GW (1998). Opioids, confusion and opioid rotation. *Palliative Medicine* **12**, 63–64

Heiskanen T & Kalso E (1997). Controlled-release oxycodone and morphine in cancer related pain. *Pain* **73**, 37–45

Houde R, Wallenstein S, Beaver W (1966). Evaluation of analgesics in patients with cancer pain. In Lasagna L (ed.) *Clinical Pharmacology*, Section 6, volume 1, *International Encyclopedia of Pharmacology and Therapeutics*. Oxford: Pergamon Press, pp 59–98

Inturrisi CE, Max MB, Foley KM, Schultz M, Shin SU, Houde RW (1984). The pharmacokinetics of heroin in patients with chronic pain. *New England Journal of Medicine* **310**, 1213–1217

Jeal W & Benfield P (1997). Transdermal fentanyl. A review of its pharmacological properties and therapeutic efficiency in pain control. *Drugs* **53**, 109–138

Kaiko RF, Wallenstein SL, Rogers AG, Grabinski PY, Houde RW (1981). Analgesic and mood effects of heroin and morphine in cancer patients with postoperative pain. *New England Journal of Medicine* **304**, 1501–1505

Kalso E, Heiskanen T, Rantio M, Rosenberg PH, Vainio A (1996). Epidural and subcutaneous morphine in the management of cancer pain: a double-blind cross-over study. *Pain* **67**, 443–449

Kirkham SR & Pugh R (1995). Opioid analgesia in uraemic patients. *The Lancet* **345**: 1185

Kissin I, Brown PT, Bradley EL Jr (1991). Magnitude of acute tolerance to opioids is not related to their potency. *Anesthesiology* **75**, 813–816

Lawlor P, Turner K, Hanson J, Bruera E (1997). Dose ratio between morphine and hydromorphone in patients with cancer pain: a retrospective study. *Pain* **72**, 79–85

Lawlor PG, Turner KS, Kanson J, Bruera ED (1998). Dose ratio between morphine and methadone in patients with cancer pain: a retrospective study. *Cancer* **82**, 1167–1173

Leng G & Finnegan MJ (1994). Successful use of methadone in nociceptive cancer pain unresponsive to morphine. *Palliative Medicine* **8**, 153–155

Ling GS, Paul D, Simantov R, Pasternak GW (1989). Differential development of acute tolerance to analgesia, respiratory depression, gastrointestinal transit and hormone release in a morphine infusion model. *Life Sciences* **45**, 1627–1636

Macdonald N, Der L, Allen S, Champion P (1993). Opioid hyperexcitability: the application of alternate opioid therapy. *Pain* **53**, 353–355

McQuay HJ, Carroll D, Faura CC, Gavaghan DJ, Hand CW, Moore RA (1990). Oral morphine in cancer pain: influences on morphine and metabolite concentration. *Clinical Pharmacology and Therapeutics* **48**, 236–244

Maddocks I, Somogyi A, Abbott F, Hayball P, Parker D (1996). Attenuation of morphine-induced delirium in palliative care by substitution with infusion of oxycodone. *Journal of Pain and Symptom Management* **12**, 182–189

Makin MK, O'Donnell V, Skinner JM, Ellershaw JE (1998). Methadone in the management of cancer related neuropathic pain. *Pain Clinics* **10**, 275–279

Martin WR, Eades CG, Thompson JA, Huppler RE, Gilbert PE (1976). The effects of morphine- and nalorphine-like drugs in the nondependent and morphine-dependent chronic spinal dog. *Journal of Pharmacology and Experimental Therapeutics* **197**, 157–132

Mercadente S, Caligara M, Sapio M, Serretta R, Lodi F (1997a). Subcutaneous fentanyl infusion in a patient with bowel obstruction and renal failure. *Journal of Pain and Symptom Management* **13**, 241–244

Mercadente S, Dardanoni G, Salvaggio L, Armata MG, Agnello A (1997b). Monitoring of opioid therapy in advanced cancer pain patients. *Journal of Pain and Symptom Management* **13**, 204–212

Morley JS (1998). Opioid rotation: does it have a role? *Palliative Medicine* **12**, 464–466

Morley JS, Watt JW, Wells JC, Miles JB, Finnegan MJ, Leng G (1993). Methadone in pain uncontrolled by morphine. *The Lancet* **342**, 1243

Moskowitz AS & Goodman RR (1985). Autoradiographic analysis of mu1 mu2 and delta opioid binding in the central nervous system of C57BL/6BY and CXBK (opioid-receptor deficient) mice. *Brain Research* **369**, 108–116

Moulin DE, Ling GS, Pasternak GW (1988). Unidirectional cross-tolerance between morphine and levorphanol in the rat. *Pain* **33**, 233–233

Osborne RJ, Joel SP, Slevin ML (1986). Morphine intoxication in renal failure: the role of morphine-6-glucuronide. *British Medical Journal* **292**, 1548–1549

Paix A, Coleman A, Lees J, Brooksbank M, Thorne D, Ashby M (1995). Subcutaneous fentanyl and sufentanil infusion substitution for morphine intolerance in cancer pain management *Pain* **63**, 263–269

Paul D, Standifer KM, Inturrisi CE, Pasternak GW (1989). Pharmacological characterization of morphine-6ß-glucuronide, a very potent morphine metabolite. *Journal of Pharmacology and Experimental Therapeutics* **251**, 477–483

Paul D, Levison JA, Howard DH, Pick CG, Hahn EF, Pasternak GW (1990). Naloxone benzoylhydrazone (NalBzoH) analgesia. *Journal of Pharmacology and Experimental Therapeutics* **255**, 769–774

Pick CG, Cheng J, Paul D, Pasternak GW (1991). Genetic influences in opioid analgesic sensitivity in mice. *Brain Research* **566**, 295–298

Portenoy RK, Payne R, Coluzzi P *et al.* (1999). Oral transmucosal fentanyl citrate (OTFC) for the treatment of breakthrough pain in cancer patients: a controlled dose titration study. *Pain* **79**, 303–312

Poyhia R, Vainio A, Kalso E (1993). A review of oxycodone's clinical pharmacokinetics and pharmacodynamics. *Journal of Pain and Symptom Management* **8**, 63–67

Ripamonti C, Groff L, Brunelli C, Polastri D, Stavrakis A, De Conno F (1998). Switching from morphine to oral methadone in treating cancer pain: what is the equianalgesic dose ratio? *Journal of Clinical Oncology* **16**, 3216–3221

Ross FB & Smith MT (1997). The intrinsic antinociceptive effects of oxycodone appear to be kappa opioid receptor mediated. *Pain* **73**, 151–157

Rossi GC, Brown GP, Leventhal L, Yang K, Pasternak GW (1996). Novel receptor mechanism for heroin and morphine-6 beta-glucuronide. *Neuroscience Letters* **216**, 1–4

Schmauss C & Yaksh TL (1984). In vivo studies on spinal opioid receptor systems mediating antinociception. II. Pharmacological profiles suggesting a differential association of mu, delta and kappa receptors with visceral, chemical and cutaneous thermal stimuli in the rat. *Journal of Pharmacology and Experimental Therapeutics* **228**, 1–12

Scholes CF, Gonty N, Trotman IF (1999). Methadone titration in opioid-resistant cancer pain. *European Journal of Cancer Care* **8**, 26–29

Schug SA, Zech D, Grond S, Jung H, Meuser T, Stobbe B (1992). A long-term survey of morphine in cancer patients. *Journal of Pain and Symptom Management* **7**, 259–266

Sindrup SH & Jensen TS (1999). Efficacy of pharmacological treatments of neuropathic pain: an update and effect related to mechanism of action. *Pain* **83**, 389–400

Sjogren P, Jonsson T, Jenssen NH, Drenck NE, Jensen TS (1993). Hyperalgesia and myoclonus in terminal cancer patients treated with continuous intravenous morphine. *Pain* **55**, 93–97

Sjogren P, Jensen NH, Jensen TS (1994). Disappearance of morphine-induced hyperalgesia after discontinuing or substituting morphine with other opioid agonists. *Pain* **59**, 313–316

Sosnowski M & Yaksh T (1990). Differential cross-tolerance between intrathecal morphine and sufentanil in the rat. *Anesthesiology* **73**, 1141–1147

Thomas Z & Bruera E (1995). Use of methadone in a highly tolerant patient receiving parenteral hydromorphone. *Journal of Pain and Symptom Management* **10**, 315–317

Trujillo KA, Akil H (1991). Inhibition of morphine tolerance and dependence by the NMDA receptor antagonist MK-801. *Science* **251**, 85–87

TTS Fentanyl Multicentre Study Group (1994). Transdermal Fentanyl in Cancer Pain. *Journal of Drug Development* **6**, 93–97

Twycross R (1998). Opioid rotation: does it have a role? *Palliative Medicine* **12**, 60–63

Vaught JL, Mathiasen JR, Raffa RB (1988). Examination of the involvement of supraspinal and spinal mu and delta opioid receptors in analgesia using the mu receptor deficient CXBT mouse. *Journal of Pharmacology and Experimental Therapeutics* **245**, 13–16

Vigano A, Fan D, Bruera E (1996). Individualized use of methadone and opioid rotation in the comprehensive management of cancer pain associated with poor prognostic indicators. *Pain* **67**, 115–119

Wall PD (1990). Neuropathic pain. *Pain* **43**, 267–268

Watanabe S, Pereira J, Hanson J, Bruera E (1998). Fentanyl by continuous subcutaneous infusion for the management of cancer pain: a retrospective study. *Journal of Pain and Symptom Management* **16**, 323–326

Watson CPN & Babul N (1998). Efficacy of oxycodone in neuropathic pain. *Neurology* **50**, 1837–1841

Woodhouse A, Ward E, Mather L (1999). Intra-subject variability in post-operative patient-controlled analgesia (PCA): is the patient equally satisfied with morphine, pethidine and fentanyl? *Pain* **80**, 545–553

World Health Organization (1986). *Cancer Pain Relief.* Geneva: WHO

World Health Organization (1996). *Cancer Pain Relief: A guide to opioid availability*, 2nd edn. Geneva: WHO

Yeh SY, Gorodetzky CW, Krebs HA (1977). Isolation and identification of morphine 3- and 6-glucuronides, morphine 3,6-diglucuronide, morphine 3-ethereal sulfate, normorphine, and normorphine 6-glucuronide as morphine metabolites in humans. *Journal of Pharmaceutical Sciences* **66**, 1288–1293

Yue QY, Svensson JO, Alm C, Sjoqvist F, Sawe J (1989). Codeine *O*-demethylation co-segregates with polymorphic debrisoquinine hydroxylation. *British Journal of Clinical Pharmacology* **28**, 639–645

Chapter 5

Scientific evidence and expert clinical opinion for the use of co-analgesics

Matthew K Makin and Jennifer Smith

Introduction

Co-analgesics, such as anticonvulsants and corticosteroids, embody a heterogeneous family of drugs that have principal indications other than as painkillers. Represented on each step of the World Health Organization (WHO) ladder, co-analgesics (the term 'adjuvant analgesics' is often used synonymously) offer help in the management of cancer pain syndromes, such as muscle spasm, and neuropathic, bone and visceral pain, which may respond poorly to combinations of opioids and non-opioids. The rationale underlying co-analgesic use is to target analgesic mechanisms involved in the generation or maintenance of pain, which enhance, or are independent of, the effects of opioids. The principle here is drug synergy, i.e. co-analgesics may allow a relatively smaller dose of opioid to be used to promote analgesia, achieving a more propitious balance between pain relief and side effects. The strategy of using opioids, non-opioids and adjuvant analgesics in combination should offer good or moderate relief of pain to about 80% of cancer patients (Zech *et al.* 1995). Portenoy (2000) suggested that co-analgesics should be grouped into four major classes according to their use: those drugs that can work for any type of pain (multipurpose analgesics), and those that are used predominantly for neuropathic, musculoskeletal or specific cancer pain syndromes (Table 5.1).

Helpful data are emerging from systematic reviews and controlled trials examining the effectiveness of co-analgesics in managing chronic non-malignant pain (McQuay *et al.* 1996; O'Malley *et al.* 2000; Wiffen *et al.* 2001). There are, however, important gaps in our knowledge about their use in cancer-related pain, even if we assume a shared, or at least a similar, pathophysiology. The picture is complicated by the fact that patients with cancer are often taking other drugs and have associated co-morbidity such as hepatic or renal impairment. These factors place cancer patients at increased risk of drug interactions or side effects.

Trials of certain co-analgesics, particularly the bisphosphonates, have focused on cancer-related pain (Lipton *et al.* 2000), but a paucity of evidence in the literature persists, and the use of many agents is still guided by personal experience and opinion. This is particularly true of the more novel co-analgesics, which may have shown a potential benefit in the laboratory or anecdotal success in small numbers of patients, and there is an understandable temptation to prescribe enthusiastically,

Table 5.1 Adjuvant analgesics: major classes

Multipurpose analgesics	Example
Steroids	Dexamethasone
Antidepressants	Amitriptyline
Neuropathic pain	
Anticonvulsants	Gabapentin
GABA agonists	Baclofen
α_2-Agonists	Clonidine
N-Methyl-D-aspartate receptor antagonists	Ketamine
Oral local anaesthetics	Mexiletene
Musculoskeletal pain	
Muscle relaxants	Baclofen
Benzodiazepines	Diazepam
Cancer pain	
Osteoclast inhibitors	Pamidronate
Radiopharmaceuticals	Strontium
Hormonal analogues	Octreotide

Modified from: Portenoy (2000).

extrapolating results from basic science and non-cancer pain directly to cancer patients.

Comprehensive assessment of the individual patient is fundamental in addressing the suffering associated with any troublesome symptom. Developing a rational approach for prescribing co-analgesics requires an understanding of the pathophysiology of pain. Familiarity with other palliative interventions for the pain syndrome is essential and the available evidence on relative benefits and burdens of any treatment must be considered. A balance is needed between the insouciant employment of unproven therapies and the desire to use only agents showing unequivocal effectiveness in double-masked, controlled trials. Often, however, it is a case of trying to do our best, employing the aristotelian virtue of 'phronesis' or sound clinical judgement.

The development of local guidelines for the use of co-analgesics, albeit well intentioned, can often lead to the unexplained variations in practice or the use of some agents before their effectiveness, or indeed their safety, has been established. Ill-conceived guidelines can be potentially dangerous, but those that have been carefully drawn up and critically appraised have been shown to improve cost-effectiveness and outcomes (Smith 2000).

Evidence-based guidelines have been developed for the use of bisphosphonates in the control of pain from bone metastases and the use of co-analgesics in cancer-related neuropathic pain by the Association for Palliative Medicine Science

Committee (Mannix *et al*. 2000) and the Mersey Palliative Care Audit Group, respectively (Figure 5.1) (Makin *et al*. 2000). In this chapter we have focused on cancer-related neuropathic pain to illustrate a cancer pain syndrome in which co-analgesics may be particularly useful.

- The WHO guidelines for cancer pain relief should be applied. Prompt referral, where appropriate, for palliative interventions such as radiotherapy or neuroanaesthetic procedures can avoid unnecessary suffering.
- In selected patients if nerve compression is suspected consider a trial of steroids if no contraindications. Use **dexamethasone** 8 mg daily for 5 days; if successful titrate down to lowest effective dose and consider suitability for radiotherapy; if ineffective after 5 days then stop.
- Consider early referral to pain specialist at any point of algorithm if pain severe.

> Amitriptyline 10 mg at night in elderly patients or 25 mg
> Increase to 100 mg if tolerated, by 25 mg every 3 days

If no response stop drug. If partial response continue and, in addition

> Trial of **anticonvulsant** if no contraindications (see Table 5.2)

If no response stop drug. If partial response continue and, in addition

> **Specialist management** (consult chronic pain specialist)

Continue if response

Figure 5.1 Pharmacological management of cancer-related neuropathic pain: an algorithm of adjuvant therapy – the Mersey Palliative Care Audit Group guidelines.

Neuropathic pain

Damage, or dysfunction, of the central or peripheral nervous system may cause neuropathic pain. Along with movement-related pain, visceral pains and pain associated with muscle spasm, neuropathic pain is disproportionately represented among patients whose pain responds poorly to morphine (Portenoy & Hagen 1990). Grond *et al*. (1999) found this to be a distressing feature of cancer pain in 213 patients (36%), in a series of 595 referred to their anaesthetic-based pain service.

Cancer-related neuropathic pain

Pain from nerve compression can occur in the early stages of plexopathy (tumour pressing on a plexus of nerves) and in radiculopathy (nerve root entrapment). Nerve compression has a nociceptive component because of stimulation of nociceptors within the nervi nervorum (the nerves supplying the nerve sheath). The pain of radiculopathy is usually in a dermatomal distribution and can be associated with objective sensory and motor signs. It is seen typically in vertebral collapse as a result of metastatic disease. Infiltration of a nerve plexus can produce several pain syndromes, depending on the pattern of nerve involvement. Cervical plexopathy is common in head and neck tumours, when pain can radiate to the ear or occiput, and is often associated with local disturbance of the sympathetic nervous system (Horner's syndrome). Brachial plexopathy can occur in apical lung tumours (Pancoast's tumour); lymph node metastases from breast carcinoma often cause pain involving the elbow, forearm, and fourth and fifth fingers. Gynaecological or colorectal carcinomas can cause lumbosacral plexopathy. Higher lesions of lumbar plexus can cause lower abdominal and thigh pain, whereas involvement of the lower plexus causes buttock and perineal pain, and bowel and bladder function may be affected. Paraneoplastic peripheral neuropathy may be associated with small cell lung cancer and is thought to be an autoimmune process.

Neuropathic pain can also complicate treatment. Chronic neuropathic pain can follow mastectomy, neck dissection and thoracotomy. Phantom pains can arise from parts of the body (typically limbs) that are surgically removed. Both early and late-onset brachial plexopathies have been described after axillary radiotherapy. Vincristine, cisplatin and paclitaxel have all been associated with painful peripheral neuropathies (Martin & Hagen 1997).

Neuropathic pain rarely localises to the precise point of damage or disruption, and patients often describe an area of pain in the distribution of the injured nerve or nerves. Sensation in the area of pain can be unpleasantly abnormal (dysaesthetic) and acutely sensitive; some patients cannot bear to be touched, even by their clothes or bedsheets. The unpleasant sensations characteristic of neuropathic pain are often associated with particular descriptive terms: paradoxical burning or 'ice burn' is virtually pathognomonic, and other descriptive terms commonly used by patients are intense aching, shooting and tingling. Sensory changes can be demonstrated clinically, and there is characteristic difficulty in distinguishing warm from cool. The clinician may be able to demonstrate allodynia, a non-painful stimulus causing pain (e.g. light touch) and hyperalgesia, which is an exaggerated response to a stimulus that is normally painful. These hypersensitisation states are characteristic of neuropathic pain.

Pathophysiology

Neuropathic pain states are maintained by complex mechanisms involving altered peripheral activity, central excitatory or inhibitory activity, and involvement of the sympathetic nervous system (Dickenson *et al.* 1997). Both physiological and neuroanatomical changes can occur. Areas within the nervous system processing pain messages appear to undergo hypersensitisation. Large peripheral nerve fibres

(Aβ-fibres) are involved in the genesis of neuropathic pain, re-organising in the dorsal horn of the spinal cord when damaged, and forming new circuits and connections. This new mesh of nerves is exquisitely sensitive and may misinterpret and amplify the input from smaller peripheral nerve (C-fibres). Sodium channels cluster at the site of peripheral nerve injury, setting up chaotic ectopic activity that results in disorganised sensory input bombarding an already sensitised dorsal horn. Disruption of nerve fibres also leads to the actual loss of opioid receptors within the nerve or its connections (Besse *et al.* 1990) and, in animal models that simulate peripheral nerve damage, a wide variety of neuropeptides and their receptors are affected which may modulate response to opioids.

Monoamines such as serotonin (Blier & Abbott 2001) and noradrenaline (Bohn *et al.* 2000) also play significant roles in descending inhibitory pathways, dampening incoming pain impulses.

Cholecystokinin (CCK) (Zhang *et al.* 2000) receptors are intimately linked to μ-opioid receptors and, when CCK binds to its receptor, the changes induced reduce the response to μ-opioid agonists such as morphine (Dertwinkel *et al.* 1999). In neuropathic pain states, work on animal models has suggested that CCK receptors are upregulated and may contribute to the relatively poor response to morphine seen in neuropathic pain (Antunes Bras *et al.* 1999).

There is also increasing evidence that neuropathic pain states involve the prolonged activation of the *N*-methyl-D-aspartate (NMDA) receptor. This leads to increased neuronal activity or 'wind up' (Coderre *et al.* 1993). In this state of hypersensitisation, mechanical and thermal stimuli are amplified, resulting in the development of hyperalgesia and allodynia. This process is thought to be mediated via the release of excitatory amino acids. γ-Aminobutyric acid (GABA) is a principal inhibitory transmitter. Stimulation of the GABA–receptor complex appears to prevent low-threshold inputs from triggering nociception (Hao *et al.* 1992), suggesting that excitatory amino acid antagonists and GABA or glycine agonists may offer therapeutic benefit.

Co-analgesics and site of action

This increased understanding of the neurobiology of neuropathic pain has encouraged new therapeutic approaches in treatment: corticosteroids, antidepressants, anticonvulsants, NMDA-receptor antagonists and GABA analogues are used as adjuvants, often in combination. There are many potential targets for co-analgesics; steroids may alleviate the inflammatory processes at the site of nerve damage and relieve nerve compression by reducing oedema. Monoamines such as noradrenaline and serotonin become deactivated after re-uptake at nerve terminals and drugs that block this re-uptake (e.g. tricyclic antidepressants) have been shown to be effective in the management of neuropathic pain. The anticonvulsants have a diverse spectrum of activity: some inhibit the genesis of chaotic peripheral ectopic activity through sodium channel blockade. Other anticonvulsants act by modulating the action of excitatory amino acids via the GABA system, or through the NDMA–receptor complex (Table 5.2). There also appears to be potential for CCK antagonists to exert an analgesic effect.

Table 5.2 Anticonvulsants as co-analgesics

As a result of the relative paucity of comparative evidence in relation to anticonvulsants, the choice of anticonvulsant will depend, to an extent, on the clinician's individual experience and preference. If in doubt, seek specialist advice.

Carbamazepine	
Mechanism of action	Slows rate of sodium channel recovery from inactivation
Side effects	Nausea, ataxia, drowsiness and confusion
Important interactions	Metabolism inhibited by erythromycin; effect of carbamazepine also enhanced by dextropropoxyphene
Dosage	Start with 100 mg daily in elderly patients or 200 mg daily; increase dose by 200 mg every 3 days until response or side effects
Sodium valproate	
Mechanism of action	Stimulates GABA synthesis, inhibits GABA degradation and also prolongs recovery of voltage-activated sodium channels
Side effects	Gastrointestinal upset, ataxia, drowsiness and hepatic impairment. Very rarely, fulminant hepatitis
Important interactions	Raises plasma levels of phenobarbital. Very rarely, absence status epilepticus when given with clonazepam
Dosage	Give 200 mg at night; increase by 200 mg every third day to maximum of 1,000 mg at night

continued...

ERRATUM
See page 63 Table 5.2. Clonazepam dosing should read 500 micrograms as starting dose, increasing by 500 microgram increments to a maximum dose of 3 milligrams.

Table 5.2 *continued...*

Clonazepam	
Mechanism of action	Enhances GABA-induced inhibitory effects
Side effects	Drowsiness and lethargy
Important interactions	As with other hypnotics and anxiolytics
Dosage	Give once at night, start at 500 mg; increase by 500 mg every third day to maximum of 3 mg; can be given via syringe driver
Gabapentin	
Mechanism of action	Gabapentin is a chemical analogue of GABA, but does not act as a GABA-receptor agonist. It binds to a receptor site in the CNS, gabapentin-binding protein, and interacts with calcium channels (Taylor *et al.* 1998). It increases GABA synthesis and release but its exact mechanism of action is still not fully understood
Side effects	Generally well tolerated, but initially somnolence ataxia and fatigue
Dosage	Start with 300 mg at night; increase after 3 days to 300 mg twice daily then to 300 mg three times a day. Increase as tolerated every third day to a maximum of 1,800 mg per day in divided doses

From Twycross *et al.* (1998) and McNamara (1996).

Why use co-analgesics in cancer-related neuropathic pain?

Some commentators believe that neuropathic pain is distinct from nociceptive pain because of its inherent insensitivity to opioids. Others have suggested that such differentation is unclear because, in practice, it is the side effects that limit escalation to an opioid dose that would promote satisfactory analgesia. This is evident from clinical trials that have reported the successful use of oxycodone (Watson & Babul 1998) and fentanyl (Dellemijn & Vanneste 1997) in neuropathic pain states.

We have described various mechanisms, some independent of opioid receptor systems, that generate or maintain pathological pain. These factors essentially push the opioid dose–response curve to the right, i.e. more drug is required to achieve analgesia. However, this higher dose may lead to the development of side effects.

By using co-analgesia to target pain-generating mechanisms and receptor complexes other than opioid systems, the 'maximal effect' (analgesia) may be achieved with a relatively smaller dose of opioid, i.e. the dose–response curve shifts back to the right.

Application in clinical practice

Neuropathic pain is a challenging pain syndrome, but it is not intractable and can be relieved by multimodal treatment following the WHO guidelines. Grond *et al.* (1999) found that the probability of successful pain relief was independent of whether patients had neuropathic components to their pain, but those with neuropathic components required more co-analgesics, notably antidepressants, anticonvulsants and corticosteroids.

The corticosteroids are useful, multipurpose co-analgesics. However, long-term use is limited by the side effects. By reducing oedema at the site of injury, they can be useful adjuvants in managing neuropathic pain caused by nerve compression. Analgesic response to corticosteroids is often viewed as a good predictor of response to radiotherapy, if indicated. In a randomised controlled trial, Vecht *et al.* (1989) found that steroids were profoundly analgesic in 37 patients with spinal cord compression, although there was no difference between conventional-dose (10 mg i.v.) and high-dose dexamethasone (100 mg i.v.) on pain.

Data, from systematic reviews on the efficacy and burdens of antidepressants as co-analgesics in chronic non-malignant pain, have been important in confirming their use in a number of neuropathic pain states. In an important systematic review of 17 randomised controlled trials, involving 10 antidepressants, the investigators concluded that, compared with placebo, of 100 patients with neuropathic pain who are given antidepressants, 30 will obtain more than 50% pain relief, 30 will have minor adverse reactions and 4 will have to stop treatment because of major adverse effects (McQuay *et al.* 1996). Comparisons of tricyclic antidepressants did not show any significant difference between them, and they were significantly more effective than benzodiazepines in the three comparisons available. Recently, there have also been reports of success using some of the more novel antidepressants that act on serotoninergic and noradrenergic systems, such as mirtazapine (Brannon & Stone 1999) and venlafaxine (Pernia 2000).

Considering the widespread use of antidepressants as co-analgesics in cancer-related pain, randomised controlled trials are conspicuous by their absence in the literature. One randomised, double-masked, placebo-controlled, cross-over trial studied the effectiveness of amitriptyline in relieving neuropathic pain after the surgical treatment of breast cancer. In this study, amitriptyline significantly relieved neuropathic pain both in the arm and around the breast scar of the patients studied (Eija *et al.* 1996).

With very similar results for anticonvulsants, it has still been unclear which drug class should be chosen first and this is often influenced by the clinician's personal preference. A recent Cochrane collaboration review has helped to resolve this dilemma (Wiffen *et al.* 2001). This work examined 23 trials of 6 anticonvulsants. However, only one of these studies considered cancer pain. The group concluded that, in chronic pain syndromes other than trigeminal neuralgia, anticonvulsants should be withheld until other interventions have been tried. They suggested that, although gabapentin is gaining increased favour in the management of neuropathic pain, the evidence suggests that it is no more effective than carbamazepine. In the study involving cancer patients, phenytoin 200 mg/day was compared with buprenorphine alone and with a combination of buprenorphine and phenytoin (100 mg/day) for treating cancer pain (Yajnik *et al.* 1992). The investigators concluded that a low dose of phenytoin was well tolerated, and the group that received combination therapy had better pain relief and significantly fewer side effects than those treated with buprenorphine alone. In an open study, Caraceni *et al.* (1999) examined the utility of gabapentin as an 'add-on' therapy to 22 patients with neuropathic cancer pain that was only partially responsive to opioid therapy; 20 patients judged the new drug to be efficacious in relieving their symptoms. In those who responded, there was a significant reduction in global pain scores and burning pain intensity; of nine patients in whom allodynia was demonstrated, the burning pain disappeared in seven during gabapentin administration.

Clonazepam is a long-acting benzodiazepine with cholinergic/GABAergic/ serotoninergic and sedative properties. In a double-masked pilot study, it has been shown to be effective in the treatment of temporomandibular joint dysfunction and associated myofascial pain (Harkins *et al.* 1991). There is also a report of effectiveness in the management of a series of patients with stomatodynia (burning mouth syndrome) (Woda *et al.* 1998). Many palliative care physicians favour clonazepam as their co-analgesic anticonvulsant of choice, pragmatically because of the once at night oral dosage schedule and its ability to be administered subcutaneously via syringe driver.

On the subject of the parenteral administration of co-analgesics, there is good evidence that clonidine, an α_2-adrenergic agonist, can be effective in managing cancer-related neuropathic pain when given via the epidural route. The Epidural Clonidine Study Group (Eisenach *et al.* 1995) studied 85 patients with severe cancer pain in whom dose-limiting side effects to morphine led to inadequate analgesia. In this double-masked, placebo-controlled trial patients were randomised to receive epidural clonidine 30 µg/h or placebo for 14 days, together with rescue epidural morphine. Successful analgesia was more common with epidural clonidine than with placebo, and this was particularly prominent in patients with neuropathic pain. Hypotension complicated clonidine therapy in two patients and in one receiving placebo.

Although intravenous lidocaine (lignocaine) has shown some benefit in a variety of chronic pain types, it has not been shown to be of any use in cancer-related

neuropathic pain (Ellemann *et al.* 1989). In a pilot study, the Eastern Cooperative Oncology Group studied 21 cancer patients who received courses of either mexiletine or flecainide (Chong *et al.* 1997). In 17 cases, there was no suggestion of benefit. Two cases had relatively clear-cut analgesic benefit and two others had some suggestion of mild-to-moderate analgesic relief. Flecainide was relatively well tolerated, but mexiletine appeared to cause nausea and/or vomiting in five of eight patients. This pilot trial suggested that systematically administered local anaesthetics relieved pain in only a minority of the patients studied with cancer pain. In the opinion of our group, the use of flecainide could not be justified because of the association with an increased incidence of sudden death (Pratt & Moye 1990). We also found that the utility of mexiletine is commonly limited by nausea and as such it is not recommended in our guidelines (Makin *et al.* 2000).

Baclofen, a $GABA_B$ analogue, acts on the GABA-receptor, principally at the spinal level, inhibiting the release of excitatory amino acids, glutamate and aspartate. It has shown to be particularly helpful in the paroxysmal pain associated with trigeminal neuralgia (Fromm 1994). It may hold some value as an adjunct in lancinating cancer-related neuropathic pain, but this has, as yet, not been proved. Side effects such as drowsiness and gastrointestinal upset, as well as the potential for a withdrawal syndrome, mean that it is generally not recommended as first-line therapy.

Ketamine, some antivirals, certain phenothiazines and a number of the *dextro*-rotatory isomers of opioids (Stringer *et al.* 2000) have been shown to have putative action at the NMDA receptor. There is increasing interest in their use in the management of neuropathic pain. Non-competitive antagonists at this receptor complex have been shown, in animal models, to block the hypersensitivity characteristic of neuropathic pain, potentiating the analgesic action and attenuating the development of tolerance to morphine (Chapman & Dickenson 1992). This marked synergy between NMDA-receptor antagonists and μ-opioid agonists has been described with the subcutaneous co-administration of ketamine in many cases of intractable cancer pain (Finlay 1999). In a randomised controlled, double-masked, cross-over, double-dose study, intravenous ketamine was shown to improve morphine analgesia in cancer-related neuropathic pain. However, drowsiness was a common side effect and a significant number of patients reported dysphoria and hallucinations (Mercadante *et al.* 2000). There have reports describing the use of oral ketamine as a co-analgesic. A recent trial followed a series of 21 patients with chronic neuropathic pain; all received an escalating dose of oral ketamine to a maximum of 100 mg. Those who showed an analgesic response were entered into a trial with integral *n*-of-1 design. Only two patients showed sufficient benefit to continue the drug beyond the end of the trial and almost half experienced unpleasant adverse effects (Haines & Gaines 1999).

Dextromethorphan, in combination with morphine (Morphidex), enhanced analgesia in a double-masked study (Katz 2000), but, when used as single agent in a variety of pain syndromes, results have been disappointing (Gilron *et al.* 2000; Plesan *et al.* 2000). Intravenous amantadine, an antiviral agent, has produced positive outcomes in cancer patients with post-surgical neuropathic pain compared with placebo. Intriguingly, a similar drug, memantine, showed potent anti-nociceptive effects in animal models (Suzuki *et al.* 2001); clinical results have, however, failed to show appreciable benefit (Eisenberg *et al.* 1998; Nikolajsen *et al.* 2000).

Conclusion

There is a bewildering number of co-analgesics for clinicians to choose from. What can be equally challenging is not so much which adjuvant to use but when to use it. Some commentators have advised maximising opioid analgesia before considering the addition of a co-analgesic (Portenoy 1998). An alternative approach is to prescribe adjuvant analgesia early on step 1 or 2 of the analgesic ladder. Either strategy is reasonable and as yet none has proved to be superior.

It is not unusual, in palliative care, to support patients undergoing potentially curative treatment through a prolonged palliative phase of illness, as well as through the terminal phase of their disease. The 'phase' of the patient's disease is rarely discussed when considering the merits or otherwise of co-analgesics. Indeed, it may be unhelpful to start certain co-analgesics in the terminal phase, where there may be considerable time lag before analgesia is achieved or when large numbers of tablets are required. We come back to sound clinical judgement, weighing the relative burdens and benefits for the individual patient in question. Certain co-analgesics (e.g. parenteral ketamine) may be appropriate for intractable pain in the terminal phase of disease, particularly when the goal may be analgesia irrespective of any sedating side effects. An approach such as this may be less desirable, as a result of the associated side effects, in treating a patient in a potentially curative phase.

When selecting co-analgesics, we must also consider the possibility of drug interactions, e.g. some antidepressants may increase the bioavailability of morphine in cancer patients (Ventafridda *et al.* 1987). Pragmatic concerns, such as drug cost, availability and the convenience of dosage regimens, can be equally important considerations.

In cancer pain management, there is a paucity of good quality evidence on the effectiveness of co-analgesics. Methodological difficulties can restrain the development of randomised controlled trials, although there are a plethora of case reports describing the benefit of individual adjuvants. Additions to the literature of anecdotal success continue, but what may be more useful are reports of the incidence and severity of adverse events associated with the use of the more novel agents.

Collectively, efforts must be concentrated on rational application of the limited evidence already available about the benefit and burden of co-analgesic use. The next step is to prioritise the gaps in our knowledge that require resolution by well-designed collaborative research.

References

Antunes Bras JM, Benoliel JJ, Bourgoin S *et al.* (1999). Effects of peripheral axotomy on cholecystokinin neurotransmission in the rat spinal cord. *Journal of Neurochemistry* **72**, 858–867

Besse D, Lombard MC, Zajac JM (1990). Pre and postsynaptic distribution of mu, delta and kappa opioid receptors in the superficial layers of the cervical dorsal horn of the rat spinal cord: a quantitative autoradiographic. *Brain Research* **521**, 15–22

Blier P & Abbott FV (2001). Putative mechanisms of action of antidepressant drugs in affective and anxiety disorders and pain. *Journal of Psychiatry and Neuroscience* **26**, 37–43

Bohn LM, Xu F, Gainetdinov RR, Caron MG (2000). Potentiated opioid analgesia in norepinephrine transporter knock-out mice. *Journal of Neuroscience* **20**, 9040–9045

Brannon GE & Stone KD (1999). The use of mirtazapine in a patient with chronic pain. *Journal of Pain and Symptom Management* **18**, 382–538

Caraceni A, Zecca E, Martini C, De Conno F (1999). Gabapentin as an adjuvant to opioid analgesia for neuropathic cancer pain. *Journal of Pain and Symptom Management* **17**, 441–445

Chapman V & Dickenson AH (1992). The combination of NMDA antagonism and morphine produces profound antinociception in the rat dorsal horn. *Brain Research* **573**, 321–323

Chong SF, Bretscher ME, Mailliard JA *et al.* (1997). Pilot study evaluating local anesthetics administered systemically for treatment of pain in patients with advanced cancer. *Journal of Pain and Symptom Management* **13** (2), 112–117

Coderre TJ, Katz J, Vaccarino AL, Melzak R (1993). Contribution of central neuroplasticity to pathological pain. *Pain* **52**, 259–285

Dellemijn PL, Vanneste JA (1997). Randomised double-blind active-placebo-controlled crossover trial of intravenous fentanyl in neuropathic pain. *The Lancet* **349**, 753–758

Dertwinkel R, Zenz M, Strumpf M, Donner B (1999). Clinical status of opioid tolerance in long-term therapy of chronic noncancer pain. In Kalso E, McQuay H, Wiesenfeld-Hallin Z (eds) *Opioid Sensitivity of Chronic Noncancer Pain*. Seattle: IASP Press, pp 129–141

Dickenson AH, Chapman V, Green GM (1997). The pharmacology of excitatory and inhibitory amino acid-mediated events in the transmission and modulation of pain in the spinal cord. *General Pharmacology* **28**, 633–638

Eija K, Tiina T, Pertti NJ (1996). Amitriptyline effectively relieves neuropathic pain following treatment of breast cancer. *Pain* **64**, 293–302

Eisenach JC, DuPen S, Dubois M, Miguel R, Allin D (1995). Epidural clonidine analgesia for intractable cancer pain. The Epidural Clonidine Study Group. *Pain* **61**, 391–399

Eisenberg E, Kleiser A, Dortort A, Haim T, Yarnitsky D (1998). The NMDA (N-methyl-D-aspartate) receptor antagonist memantine in the treatment of postherpetic neuralgia: a double-blind, placebo-controlled study. *European Journal of Pain* **2**, 321–327

Ellemann K, Sjogren P, Banning AM, Jensen TS, Smith T, Geertsen P (1989). Trial of intravenous lidocaine on painful neuropathy in cancer patients. *Clinical Journal of Pain* **5**, 291–294

Finlay I (1999). Ketamine and its role in cancer pain. *Pain Reviews* **6**, 303–313

Fromm GH (1994). Baclofen as an adjuvant analgesic. *Journal of Pain and Symptom Management* **9**, 500–509

Gilron I, Booher SL, Rowan MS, Smoller MS, Max MB (2000). A randomized, controlled trial of high-dose dextromethorphan in facial neuralgias. *Neurology* **55**, 964–971

Grond S, Radbruch L, Meuser T, Sabatowski R, Loick G, Lehmann KA (1999). Assessment and treatment of neuropathic cancer pain following WHO guidelines. *Pain* **79**, 15–20

Haines DR, Gaines SP (1999). N of 1 randomised controlled trials of oral ketamine in patients with chronic pain. *Pain* **83**, 283–287

Hao JX, Xu XJ, Yu YX, Seiger A, Wiesenfeld-Hallin Z (1992). Baclofen reverses the hypersensitivity of dorsal horn wide dynamic range neurons to mechanical stimulation after transient spinal cord ischemia; implications for a tonic GABAergic inhibitory control of myelinated fiber input. *Journal of Neurophysiology* **68**, 392–396

Harkins S, Linford J, Cohen J, Kramer T, Cueva L (1991). Administration of clonazepam in the treatment of TMD and associated myofascial pain: a double-blind pilot study. *Journal of Craniomandibular Disorders* **5**, 179–186

Katz N (2000). MorphiDex: double-blind, multiple-dose studies in chronic pain patients. *Journal of Pain and Symptom Management* **19**(suppl), 37–41

Lipton A, Theriault RL, Hortobagyi GN *et al.* (2000). Pamidronate prevents skeletal complications and is effective palliative treatment in women with breast carcinoma and osteolytic bone metastases: long term follow-up of two randomized, placebo-controlled trials. *Cancer* **88**, 1082–1090

McNamara J (1996). Drugs Effective in the therapy of the epilepsies. In Hardman & Limbird (eds) *Goodman and Gilman's The Pharmacological Basis of Therapeutics*, 9th edn. New York: McGraw-Hill

McQuay HJ, Tramer M, Nye BA, Carroll D, Wiffen PJ, Moore RA (1996). A systematic review of antidepressants in neuropathic pain. *Pain* **68**, 217–227

Makin MK, Smith J, Thompson A, Littlewood C, Skinner J, Ellershaw JE (2000). The multi-modal approach to cancer related neuropathic pain leads to improved pain control without excessive drowsiness: An open, multi-centre prospective study. *Palliative Medicine* **14**, 235 (Research abstract)

Mannix K, Ahmedzai SH, Anderson H, Bennett M, Lloyd-Williams M, Wilcock A (2000). Using bisphosphonates to control the pain of bone metastases: evidence-based guidelines for palliative care. *Palliative Medicine* **14**, 455–461

Martin LA & Hagen NA (1997). Neuropathic pain in cancer patients: mechanisms, syndromes, and clinical controversies. *Journal of Pain and Symptom Management* **14**, 99–117

Mercadante S, Arcuri E, Tirelli W, Casuccio A (2000). Analgesic effect of intravenous ketamine in cancer patients on morphine therapy: a randomized, controlled, double-blind, crossover, double-dose study. *Journal of Pain and Symptom Management* **20**, 246–252

Nikolajsen L, Gottrup H, Kristensen AG, Jensen TS (2000). Memantine (a N-methyl-D-aspartate receptor antagonist) in the treatment of neuropathic pain after amputation or surgery: a randomized, double-blinded, cross-over study. *Anesthesia and Analgesia* **91**, 960–966

O'Malley PG, Balden E, Tomkins G, Santoro J, Kroenke K, Jackson JL (2000). Treatment of fibromyalgia with antidepressants: a meta-analysis. *Journal of General Internal Medicine* **15**, 659–666

Pernia A, Mico JA, Calderon E, Torres LM (2000). Venlafaxine for the treatment of neuropathic pain. *Journal of Pain and Symptom Management* **19**, 408–410

Plesan A, Sollevi A, Segerdahl M (2000). The N-methyl-D-aspartate-receptor antagonist dextromethorphan lacks analgesic effect in a human experimental ischemic pain model. *Acta Anaesthesiologica Scandinavica* **44**, 924–928

Portenoy RK (1998). Adjuvant analgesics in pain management. In Doyle D, Hanks GW, MacDonald N (eds) *The Oxford Textbook of Palliative Medicine*, 2nd edn. Oxford: Oxford Medical Publications, 361–390

Portenoy RK (2000). Current pharmacotherapy of chronic pain *Journal of Pain and Symptom Management*. **19**(suppl 1), S16–S20

Portenoy RK & Hagen NA (1990). Breakthrough pain: definition, prevalence and characteristics. *Pain* **41**, 273–281

Pratt CM & Moye LA (1990). The Cardiac Arrhythmia Suppression Trial: background, interim results and implications. *American Journal of Cardiology* **65**(4), 20B–29B

Smith WR (2000). Evidence for the effectiveness of techniques To change physician behavior. *Chest* **118**(suppl 2), 8S–17S

Stringer M, Makin MK, Miles J, Morley JS (2000). *d*-Morphine, but not *l*-morphine, has low micromolar affinity for the non-competitive N-methyl-D-aspartate site in rat forebrain. Possible clinical implications for the management of neuropathic pain. *Neuroscience Letters* **295** (1–2), 21–24

Suzuki R, Matthews EA, Dickenson AH (2001). Comparison of the effects of MK-801, ketamine and memantine on responses of spinal dorsal horn neurones in a rat model of mononeuropathy. *Pain* **91**, 101–109

Taylor CP, Gee NS, Su TZ *et al*. (1998). A summary of mechanistic hypotheses of gabapentin pharmacology. *Epilepsy Research* **29**, 233–249

Twycross R, Wilcock A, Thorp S (1998). *Palliative Care Formulary*, 1st edn. Oxford: Radcliffe Medical Press

Vecht CJ, Haaxma-Reiche H, van Putten WL, de Visser M, Vries EP, Twijnstra A (1989). Initial bolus of conventional versus high-dose dexamethasone in metastatic spinal cord compression. *Neurology* **39**, 1255–1257

Ventafridda V, Ripamonti C, De Conno F, Bianchi M, Pazzuconi F, Panerai AE (1987). Antidepressants increase bioavailability of morphine in cancer patients. *The Lancet* **i**, 1204

Watson CP & Babul N (1998). Efficacy of oxycodone in neuropathic pain: a randomized trial in postherpetic neuralgia. *Neurology* **50**, 1837–1841

Wiffen P, Collins S, McQuay H, Carroll D, Jadad A, Moore A (2001). Anticonvulsant drugs for acute and chronic pain (Cochrane Review). In *The Cochrane Library*, vol. 1. Oxford: Update Software

Woda A, Navez ML, Picard P, Gremeau C, Pichard-Leandri E (1998). A possible therapeutic solution for stomatodynia (burning mouth syndrome). *Journal of Orofacial Pain* **12**, 272–278

Yajnik S, Singh GP, Singh G, Kumar M (1992). Phenytoin as a coanalgesic in cancer pain. *Journal of Pain and Symptom Management* **7**, 209–213

Zech DF, Grond S, Lynch J, Hertel D, Lehmann KA (1995). Validation of World Health Organization Guidelines for cancer pain relief: a 10-year prospective study. *Pain* **63**, 65–76

Zhang X, de Araujo Lucas G, Elde R, Wiesenfeld-Hallin Z, Hokfelt T (2000). Effect of morphine on cholecystokinin and mu-opioid receptor-like immunoreactivities in rat spinal dorsal horn neurons after peripheral axotomy and inflammation. *Neuroscience* **95**, 197–207

Chapter 6

Scientific evidence and expert clinical opinion for the use of medications beyond their licence

Sam Hjelmeland Ahmedzai, Mike Bennett and Colin Hardman

Introduction

Palliative medicine is based on three major principles: expert symptom control, which should be evidence based wherever possible; holistic care of the patient with advanced, ultimately fatal illness; and multidisciplinary team working. Symptom control is made easier and more effective in palliative care by the last two principles, because holistic assessment of the patient's psychosocial and spiritual needs alongside physical distress frequently identifies non-medical avenues of management, and the contributions by other members of the palliative care team are often essential to good assessment and intervention. However, the role of medical management of symptoms, and of pharmacological treatments in particular, is paramount. It is disquieting, then, to reflect that a large part of the practice of palliative medicine is based only partly on evidence, and the actual prescribing of many of the agents used in symptom control is not strictly justifiable. Furthermore, the legal basis of this prescribing is, at first sight, often on the borderline of, or frankly outwith, the current licensing arrangements in the UK. This chapter explores the reasons for these disconcerting observations, tries to clarify the practical legal issues, and proposes a framework for further discussions within the speciality of palliative medicine and related professional groups.

To tackle this complex subject rationally, this chapter tackles the following questions:

- What are UK drug-licensing regulations?
- What do we know about prescribing outside of licences in other areas of medicine?
- How does the prescribing of drugs in palliative medicine relate to the regulations?
- Why may prescribing beyond licence be harmful to patients?
- What are the rights and responsibilities of patients and carers?
- What are the duties and contributions of pharmacists?
- What is the role of nurses in palliative care prescribing?
- How can palliative medicine develop a long-term plan for rationalising its drug prescribing?

UK drug-licensing regulations

The Medicines Control Agency (MCA) is the executive arm of the UK government body responsible for regulating the pharmaceutical sector and implementing policy in this area. It defines a medicine (on the website) as follows:

> A human medicine is defined in European legislation as a product for the treatment and prevention of disease; for administration to make medical diagnosis; or for restoring, correcting or modifying physiological functions in human beings . . . .

> Medicines come in a variety of pharmaceutical forms depending on the condition to be treated and the way in which this may be done. For example, solid dosage forms such as lozenges, pastilles, tablets, pills and capsules can be designed to dissolve slowly in the mouth; or more rapidly in the stomach for better absorption or to pass through the stomach to dissolve lower in the gut; or to give a controlled release of medicament throughout the gut.

> External forms of medication include lotions, creams, ointments, liniments and skin patches. Aerosols can provide medication topically to the lungs for the rapid relief of asthma; suitable drops can carry medicaments to the eyes, ears and nose. Specially designed solid dose forms such as pessaries and suppositories carry medication into the vagina and rectum. Injections may be used to introduce medication through the skin into blood vessels or to subcutaneous tissues, muscles and other tissues in the body.

> The purpose of these various forms of medication is to carry the active constituent (the drug) to the area where it is most needed and in so doing to avoid, or keep to a minimum, any unwanted effects on other areas of the body.

The MCA's primary objective is to safeguard public health by ensuring that all medicines on the UK market meet appropriate standards of safety, quality and efficacy. The safeguarding of public health is achieved largely through a system of licensing and subsequent monitoring of medicines after they have been licensed. Medical, pharmaceutical and scientific staff of the MCA, working in multidisciplinary functional teams, assess the scientific data supplied by an applicant for a product licence (or *marketing authorisation* to use current EC terminology).

It is interesting to note that governmental regulation of medicines in England started officially during the reign of King Henry VIII (1491–1547), through fellows appointed by the Royal College of Physicians. In Scotland, the Charter from King James VI, which initiated the Royal College of Physicians and Surgeons of Glasgow in 1599, also gave it powers to inspect and control the sale of drugs. It is suggested that state control of medicines goes back even further to ancient Egyptian and Greek times, and was active in early Muslim culture (Penn 1979). In recent times the need to tighten controls on the pharmaceutical industry was dramatically highlighted by the thalidomide disaster of the 1960s, and this directly led to new legislation and the setting up in 1963 of the Committee on Safety of Drugs and later the Committee on Safety of Medicines.

In 1972 the UK government first introduced a system of licensing for medicines, whereby manufacturers needed to supply scientific data on efficacy and safety before being allowed to market a drug. This system of licensing has been influenced by EC legislation and the latter now takes precedence over UK law on this topic.

How are drugs licensed?

The main types of licences and certificates granted by the authorities that are relevant to professionals in palliative care are marketing authorisations (MAs), parallel imports product licences (PIPLs), and the clinical trial certificate (CTC). When we talk of a drug being 'licensed' or 'unlicensed', we usually mean whether or not it has an MA (or, in older UK terminology, a product licence). The PIPL covers drugs that are imported for sale into the UK from other EC countries and must be subject to the same licensing restrictions as in the originating country. The CTC is granted as part of the clinical trial exemption scheme (CTX), for new drugs being tested in phase 2 or phase 3 studies.

There are two other main types of exemptions to the above regulations: the manufacture and supply of unlicensed relevant medicinal products for individual patients ('specials') and the herbal remedies exemption. These would not normally affect a professional working in palliative care; further details on them are available at the website of the MCA.

For the purposes of clinicians, it is the marketing authorisation that is of most relevance because it allows the company holding it to: sell, supply or export a medicinal product; procure the sale, supply or export the product; procure the manufacture or assembly (i.e. packaging and labelling) of the product for sale, supply or export; or import the product. The MCA carries out pre-marketing assessment of the medicine's safety, quality and efficacy, examining all the research and test results in detail, before a decision is made on whether the product should be granted a marketing authorisation.

A company applying for an MA needs to be very precise about several key aspects of the properties of the drug, including main effects, side effects, contraindications and interactions. Sometimes a drug is granted a product licence for a very specific clinical indication, such as cytotoxics to be used only in cancer patients with a stated primary type. In other situations, the licence may cover the use of the drug for symptom control in a wide variety of diagnoses. In the field of pain control, many of the analgesics currently licensed obtained their MAs on the basis of data in chronic non-malignant pain study populations. The present product licences therefore do not strictly cover their subsequent use in patients with pain arising from cancer. Whether this actually represents a problem will be considered in more detail below, but in legal terms this distinction should be acknowledged.

A term that is often used in this area is 'off-label'. This is a general expression that covers any of the several ways that a licensed drug may be prescribed in its original (licensed) form, so that it allows the use to fall outside of the MA or product licence. Thus, a drug that holds an MA for use by the intravenous route, but which is then given to a patient by the subcutaneous route, is strictly speaking being applied 'off-label'. This is even if the drug itself is a *bona fide* licensed medicine for the present indication, e.g. morphine for the control of pain. In this way, most drugs that are be officially licensed for a specific situation can come to be used in many 'off-label' ways.

'Off-label' use is in contrast to an 'unlicensed' use of a drug, in which a drug is given that has not yet been given a licence, or has been specially imported, or if a chemical is given as a drug. Another common type of unlicensed use is when the drug is given in such a way that it no longer applies to the original, licensed situation, e.g. if a drug has a licence as an oral tablet formulation, but this is then crushed to be made into a liquid suspension, the properties of the drug may be drastically changed and the new prescription is clearly unlicensed. This is common practice in paediatrics, as will be shown below, and is also often relevant to palliative care. Table 6.1 summarises the circumstances in which a drug may be prescribed in an off-label or unlicensed fashion.

Table 6.1 Types of prescribing situations in relation to product licences in palliative medicine

	Example
Fully within licence	Oral morphine preparation given orally for pain Gabapentin given for neuropathic pain
Off-label	Oral morphine given for dyspnoea Intravenous morphine preparation given subcutaneously Amitriptyline given for neuropathic pain
Unlicensed	Oral morphine tablet given via rectal route Transdermal fentanyl patch cut in half or taped over to give lower dose

It may seem surprising that drugs that are used extensively off-label or in an unlicensed way (as the studies detailed below will show) continue to be used without a licence. It is the responsibility of the manufacturer or marketer of the drug to apply for a new licence or extension to a licence. MAs have to be renewed every 5 years, but to generate and submit new data to support an *extension* to an existing licence can be very expensive. Once a drug is out of the restriction of its original patent and is therefore copied by generic manufacturers, there is little incentive for any company to pay for the work of obtaining a new or extended licence. Thus, manufacturers may be well aware of the off-label and unlicensed use of their drugs, but may not be inclined to apply for extensions, and cannot in any of their literature make recommendations regarding these uses. A notable exception to this is the recent extensions to the licences for proton pump inhibitors, which have contributed to their rapidly increased prescription and are hugely profitably for manufacturers, even of so-called 'me-too' drugs (Bashford *et al.* 1998).

Ferner (1996) has proposed a classification of the various ways that drugs could be used beyond licence, based on several factors that describe the 'perceived reasonableness' of the practice:

- the type of patient (ranging from young adults to women in early pregnancy)
- the severity of the illness (life threatening to trivial)
- the known adverse effects of the drug
- the quality of the published data (ranging from recommended in standard textbooks to anecdotal or no published data).

It should be stressed that, in British law, both types of practice – off-label use and unlicensed use – are not illegal, but they may place the prescriber at a greater degree of risk of a formal complaint if something should go wrong. The legal responsibilities are discussed below.

In summary, a drug should normally be prescribed only in strict accordance with its marketing authorisation, which covers a particular clinical situation and indication, route, dose and frequency, and declares what is known about the expected side effects and interactions. However, in real-life clinical practice in many disciplines, including palliative medicine, a prescriber may wish to offer the same drug to a patient who does not fall into the licensed scenario. In this case, the drug can be prescribed but it is 'off-label'. Alternatively, the prescriber may wish to use an established drug in a novel way that is unlicensed. The literature that covers these kinds of use is reviewed below.

Off-label and unlicensed prescribing in other disciplines

An American questionnaire-based study conducted into the prescribing patterns of 251 physicians revealed that 88% of the respondents used drugs for off-label situations (Serradell & Galle 1993). Nearly a quarter prescribed off-label on a daily basis. In the USA, prescribing off-label may have major financial implications for the doctor or the managed-care setting, if the prescription does not comply with Food and Drug Agency (FDA) regulations. In the UK and many other European countries, there may not necessarily be financial consequences, but the clinical responsibilities are just as acute.

A discipline in which prescribing beyond the licence is apparently common is paediatrics, according to several recent studies. One involved the detailed prospective recording of drugs prescribed over a 13-week period in a medical and surgical ward in Alder Hey Children's Hospital in Liverpool (Turner *et al.* 1998). A total of 609 patients had 707 admissions during the data collection, with ages ranging from 4 days to 20 years. Altogether, 2,013 prescriptions were made out for these patients, who received between 0 and 21 different drugs. The median number of drugs they received was two on the surgical ward and one on the medical ward.

In 506 (25%) of the prescriptions, the drugs were being used in either an unlicensed (139) or off-label manner (367). These proportions were roughly similar on the medical and surgical wards. Many instances of off-label or unlicensed prescribing arise in paediatrics because the original data submitted for the MA were derived from adults. An example of off-label prescription is therefore the use of morphine, which has been licensed for intravenous administration in children aged 12 years or older, but is then used in younger patients. In this study, morphine was the fourth most commonly off-label prescribed medicine, but paracetamol was the first and another analgesic, diclofenac sodium, was third.

Turner *et al.* (1998) give interesting insights on the reasons why drugs were prescribed beyond their licences, e.g. in the surgical ward where there were 235 off-label prescriptions out of a total of 1,053, the reasons being:

* used in child of inappropriate age (130 prescriptions)
* used for different indication from that licensed (86 prescriptions)
* different dose used (nine prescriptions)
* different route of administration (nine prescriptions)
* used when contraindicated (one prescription).

As stated above, a smaller number (139) of prescriptions were for *unlicensed uses*, and these included, in the medical ward, out of a total of 960 prescriptions:

* special formulations of a licensed drug (30 prescriptions)
* modification to a licensed drug (16 prescriptions)
* new drug made available under special manufacturing licence (11 prescriptions)
* drug made from raw material (10 prescriptions)
* drug imported from another country where it is licensed but not in UK (four prescriptions)
* chemical used as a drug (three prescriptions)
* one prescription for a patient taking part in a clinical trial.

A larger study was more recently undertaken to examine off-label and unlicensed paediatric drug prescribing in five European countries (Conroy *et al.* 2000). Data were collected prospectively on prescriptions made in children's wards of five hospitals in England, Sweden, Germany, Italy and the Netherlands. Data collection in this study ran for a shorter time, namely 4 weeks. A total of 624 children were included, with ages ranging from 4 days to 16 years. They received 2,262 drug prescriptions, with a mean number of 3.6 prescriptions per patient.

Both off-label and unlicensed prescribing were common in all countries. Overall, two-thirds (67%) of the children received such a prescription during their hospital stay. There were, again, more prescriptions for off-label use (872 or 39% of all prescriptions) than for unlicensed use (164 or 7% of all prescriptions). Analgesics and bronchodilators were the most common categories of drugs used off-label. It is interesting to note that only in the British hospital was morphine in the top five of all prescriptions, whereas paracetamol came overall top in four of five countries. In the UK, morphine was also the third most common drug overall to be prescribed off-label. Conroy *et al.* (2000) found that the most common reason across all countries for off-label prescribing was deviations in dose and frequency from the original licence (accounting for 32% of prescriptions in the British hospital). Other reasons, in descending order as prescribed in the UK, were: age (39%); indication (17%); and route (12%). Deviations in formulation did not occur in this study in the UK, but were very common in the Netherlands, where they accounted for 58% of their off-label prescriptions.

The French pattern of paediatric prescribing was reported in a separate study by Chalumeau *et al.* (2000). A different methodology was used by them, in which 95 paediatricians working in Paris were asked to record all their prescriptions for patients under the age of 15 years, for 1 day. Of a total of 2,522 prescriptions administered to 989 patients, 29% were used off-label and 4% in an unlicensed way. Overall, 56% of their patients received one or more off-label prescriptions. In Israel, a retrospective analysis of medical records showed remarkably consistent results to the previous prospective studies (Gavrilov *et al.* 2000). The analysis covered 132 paediatric outpatients attending one centre over 2 months, who were aged from 1 month to 19 years: 42% of these received a prescription that was off-label or for an unlicensed medication. Of the 222 prescriptions given out, 26% were off-label and 8% were unlicensed. The most common reasons for off-label prescriptions were different dose and age from the product licences. In all cases, the unlicensed medications were modifications of licensed drugs, namely tablets that had been crushed to prepare oral suspensions.

A view from general practice came from another UK study, again focusing on prescribing patterns for children. McIntyre *et al.* (2000) conducted a retrospective analysis of all prescriptions over 1 year, for children aged 12 years and under, in a single practice in the English Midlands. During 1997 there were 3,347 prescriptions involving 1,175 children and 160 different drugs. A total of 2,828 (85%) prescriptions were covered by product licences; 11% (351) were off-label and 10 (<1%) were for unlicensed medications. In 158 (5%) prescriptions, there was insufficient information to classify the prescription.

Table 6.2 gives a summary of findings about off-label and unlicensed prescribing in published paediatric studies.

Moving away from the paediatric population, another retrospective UK study of GP prescribing by Bashford *et al.* (1998) has investigated the reasons why patients are given proton pump inhibitors (PPIs). This team used existing general practice databases from 1991 and 1995 to build up a picture of the changing patterns of PPI prescription, in relation to the changing licensed indications for this class of drug. In 1991 the most common reason was oesophagitis (which was in fact the first licensed indication), but this fell to third place in 1995. Instead, non-ulcer dysplasia now became the most common, followed by hiatus hernia and reflux. This occurred despite the fact that non-ulcer dysplasia did not become a licensed indication until 1997. The authors point out that their study included a range of PPIs, which did not share the same licensed indications, and this may have in fact under-estimated the number of off-label prescriptions.

Another professional discipline which has been studied is psychiatry. Lowe-Ponsford and Baldwin (2000) conducted a retrospective postal survey of prescribing with 200 psychiatrists. With a 58% response rate, they found that 76 respondents (65%) had prescribed off-label medication within the past month. They point out that, apart from the use of high-dose neuroleptics, there are no formal guidelines to assist psychiatrists in this area.

Prescribing outside the licence in palliative medicine

Compared with the studies described above in other disciplines, notably paediatrics, there is a paucity of quantitative data on this subject in the field of palliative medicine. The first prospective audit of actual prescribing was published by Atkinson and Kirkham (1999). Although their research was carried out in a single British 10-bedded specialist unit, they provide a useful starting point to examine prescribing practice in this speciality. Prescriptions were analysed for 76 patients, who all had advanced malignant disease, during a 4-month period. Altogether, there were 689 prescriptions, involving 84 different drugs used for the management of 34 symptoms. Two-thirds (68%) of prescriptions were for drugs and indications fully covered by their licences. Off-label prescriptions accounted for 17%, whereas the remaining 15% were unlicensed for the reason they were prescribed. The authors described these deviations beyond licence using a modified version of the classification proposed by Ferner (1996).

In palliative care, it is often necessary to administer drugs by non-oral routes, because of the frequency in this population of nausea, vomiting, dysphagia and reduced conscious level, particularly as death approaches. In this survey, 58% of prescriptions were for drugs given orally, 36% for the subcutaneous route and 5% for other routes. Of the drugs given fully in accordance with the licence, 70% were given orally, 24% subcutaneously and the remaining 6% by other routes. In contrast, the

Table 6.2 Summary of findings in paediatric studies of prescribing beyond licence

	Turner et al. (1998)	Conroy et al. (2000)	Chalumeau et al. (2000)	Gavrilov et al. (2000)	McIntyre et al. (2000)
Design	Prospective survey of drug charts	Prospective survey of drug charts	Prospective physician survey	Retrospective audit of medical records	Retrospective audit of prescriptions
Countries	England	Five EC countries	France	Israel	England
Setting	Inpatients	Inpatients	Several	Outpatients	General practice
Centres	1	5	Several	1	1
Timespan	13 weeks	4 weeks	1 day	2 months	1 year
Participants	609	624	989	132	1,175
Age range	4 days–20 years	4 days–16 years	< 15 years	1 month–19 years	< 12 years
Prescriptions	2,013	2,262	2,522	222	3,347
Off-label (%)	18	39	29	26	11
Unlicensed (%)	7	7	4	8	< 1
Unclassified (%)	–	–	–	–	5
Total beyond licence (%)	25	46	33	34	12
Patients who received medication beyond licence (%)	NA	67	56	42	NA

subcutaneous route was the most common for off-label prescriptions (54%), followed by oral (44%) and other routes (2%). This pattern was accentuated for drugs given in an unlicensed way – subcutaneous in 75%, oral in 22% and other routes in 3%. Thus, it seems that the further the prescribing is from the product licence, the more likely it is for the subcutaneous route to be used.

Atkinson and Kirkham (1999) have helpfully given further breakdowns of their prescriptions, allowing us greater insight into how off-label and unlicensed prescribing occurs. The most common reason for a prescription was pain, accounting for 28%. Of these, 80% were within the licence, 15% were off-label and 5% were unlicensed. Examples of the last category were midazolam, diazepam and dothiepin for neuropathic pain, and dexamethasone for the treatment of pain, allegedly by reduction of peritumoral oedema. There is no research to support any of these treatments, although they are commonly recommended in palliative care texts. After pain, the second most common reason for a prescription was management of agitation, insomnia or anxiety (21%). Here, 41% of prescriptions were given within the licence, another 41% off-label and as much as 18% in an unlicensed way. The last included the use of morphine elixir, diamorphine and hyoscine hydrobromide.

The management of nausea and vomiting was the third most common category of prescribing (14%), and for this drugs were given mainly within the licence (86%), whereas 11% were given off-label and in 3% an unlicensed medication was used. This medication was octreotide, which is frequently used in palliative care for the management of symptoms of intestinal obstruction in view of its known anti-secretory properties, but for which no licence exists.

All prescriptions for constipation and for infection were made within the product licences of the drugs used. With respect to dyspnoea, which surprisingly only accounted for 2.5% of all prescriptions, 47% of prescriptions were within the drugs' licences and 53% were unlicensed. The latter included nabilone, dexamethasone, midazolam, morphine and diamorphine – all of which are not licensed for this indication but have varying amounts of published research evidence for their use, and have been recommended in major palliative medicine texts (Ahmedzai 1998).

After the publication of the study by Atkinson and Kirkham (1999), a letter was published with similar data from another single UK specialist inpatient unit by Todd and Davies (1999). They found over a 6-month period, which resulted in 120 admissions, that 1,004 prescriptions were made. Of these, 15% were prescribed off-label and 12% of prescriptions were for unlicensed situations. A further 2% of prescriptions were made under a CTX arrangement or a dentists' exemption certificate (DDX).

Todd and Davies (1999) made the point that the rates of prescribing by different routes varied between their study and that of Atkinson and Kirkham (1999). In particular, their rate of use of the subcutaneous route was nearly half that of the earlier study – 20% compared with 36%. Furthermore, the second study found a higher rate of prescribing of co-analgesics. Thus they rightly identify that each study has to be carefully assessed with respect to its patient population, and the local patterns of clinical practice. For this reason, it is sad to reflect that so far there has been no multicentre prospective research to examine palliative medicine prescribing.

Why may prescribing beyond licence be harmful to patients?

In the studies described above, the published data mainly related to the frequency and reasons for prescribing beyond the drugs' licences. Do such practices necessarily mean that patients are at risk of being harmed? First, let us look at the evidence from paediatrics. Turner *et al.* (1999) investigated the relationship of adverse drug reactions (ADRs) to off-label and unlicensed prescriptions. From a 13-week surveillance of five paediatric wards in a British children's hospital, they found that 4,455 courses of drugs were administered to 936 patients during 1,046 admissions. In 507 (48%) of these admissions, patients received one or more drugs that were prescribed off-label or in an unlicensed way. ADRs occurred in 116 (11%) of the admissions. ADRs were associated with 112 (4%) of the 2,881 fully licensed prescriptions, but with 95 (6%) of the 1,574 off-label or unlicensed medications. Thus, it was concluded that prescribing beyond licence could potentially put patients at greater risk.

Clarkson *et al.* (2001) continued this theme by studying a new scheme for the reporting of ADRs to the prescription of drugs to children in the Trent region of the UK. This was a pilot for a paediatric regional monitoring centre (PRMC), which operates as an extension to the UK's current spontaneous ADR reporting scheme, based on the use of 'Yellow Cards'. During the first year of the PRMC, 95 reports of ADR were received in contrast to 40 in the previous year; 24 (25%) of these were for medications that were prescribed off-label and 26 (15%) of the ADRs were considered medically significant.

Ironically, the drug that initiated much of the current legislation on medication, thalidomide, has recently been gradually reintroduced for an increasing number of clinical indications. The largest body of published evidence is around its effectiveness in suppressing erythema nodosum in leprosy, and the FDA has approved it for this clinical situation. However, because of its known marked activity against tumour necrosis factor (TNF), thalidomide has been investigated and experimentally used for other situations, including inflammatory or immune conditions, malignancies and – relevant to palliative care – the management of cancer-related cachexia.

Clark *et al.* (2001) have reported from the USA on the first 18 months of post-marketing surveillance of oral thalidomide, in which 1,210 spontaneous reports of ADRs were made. These covered both licensed and off-label uses of the drug. Most of the ADRs to thalidomide were predictable, given the known properties of the drug, but other disturbing reports were for seizures and Stevens–Johnson syndrome. With cancer patients, there appears to be an increased risk of thalidomide-related ADRs, including thromboembolic events. The potential benefits to palliative care, which may be substantial with very distressing symptoms, must be balanced against these emerging dangers.

Apart from the induction of specific ADRs, the uncritical use of drugs beyond their licence has other potential risks. It could theoretically be a problem, e.g. where patients are expected to die in a short time, off-label or unlicensed medications may lead to an even shorter survival. This potential risk can arise with the use of combinations of opioid analgesics, neuroleptic antiemetics and often also benzodiazepine sedatives in syringe drivers for subcutaneous infusion. The fact that such regimens have not been subjected to randomized controlled trials may be understandable on one level, because of the difficulty of conducting such research in an imminently terminal population, but it does not remove the possibility that, in some patients, survival may be inadvertently shortened. The principle of double effect, in which harm may be done to a patient as an unavoidable secondary effect in the pursuit of a significant benefit elsewhere (usually control of extreme symptoms), allows for the excuse of this practice in the eyes of the law. However, it does not excuse the profession from seeking better, and more evidence-based, ways of achieving the same benefit.

Another problem is the ease with which doctors in the UK may prescribe drugs in an unmonitored way, which could in turn lead to a careless and potentially dangerous attitude. A culture in which doctors can prescribe unlicensed medication in this way, without prior consultation and monitoring by peers, is unhealthy for both the medical profession and clearly for some patients' welfare. These themes are discussed below in the context of clinical governance.

What are the legal responsibilities?

The primary medicolegal issues raised by the use of drugs, either off-label or in an unlicensed way, relate to consent from patients and the legal defence of the doctor's practice. Consent is legally valid if given by a person who is adequately informed, acting voluntarily and competent to decide (i.e. understands the information, retains and believes it, and uses it to reach a reasoned conclusion). In situations where consent cannot be given under these criteria, treatment can be given only for conditions needing immediate treatment (the doctrine of necessity). In such situations, less urgent or more unconventional treatments need the guidance of the court to declare that treatment would not be unlawful. In all cases, specific consent should be sought for use of new drugs or drugs used innovatively.

Patients can be expected to give consent only if they have received sufficient information. Doctors should inform patients about the medicines they are prescribing for at least two reasons. First, they are obliged to give information as part of their general duty of care to the patient. A doctor's failure to inform could be held to be a breach of duty which, if it causes the patient injury, renders the doctor liable to a claim for compensation. Second, patients have a right to information as part of their right to self-determination. The UK Patient's Charter underlines this principle (Anonymous 1994).

The failure to warn patients is a common cause for complaint and in the UK forms the basis for most legal claims against doctors relating to the supply of medicines. It is not always clear how much information and advice should be given and who should decide. Under English law the decision is left to doctors, but under the Patient's Charter it is the patient who decides. By legal precedent:

> . . . a doctor is not guilty of negligence if he has acted in accordance with a practice accepted as proper by a responsible body of medical men skilled in that particular art.
>
> *Bolam v Friern Hospital Management Committee* 1957

Specific consent is therefore unlikely to be necessary in the eyes of a court for off-label prescriptions that are well established and used regularly and widely for that purpose by a prescriber's peers in the field.

Not infrequently, the patient may choose *not* to be told the full details of the treatment being suggested, while still consenting to receive it. This is probably very common in palliative care, where patients may be either too ill or psychologically unwilling to enter into detailed discussions with their professional carers about medical details. Such 'uninformed consent' could be regarded as valid as long as the patient has been given the option of receiving the information (Anonymous 2001).

Moreover English law deems that the provision of *too much information* about the risks of treatment can work against a patient's best interests because:

> . . . a patient may make an unbalanced judgment if he is provided with too much information and is made aware of possibilities which he is not capable of assessing because of his lack of medical training, his prejudice or his personality
>
> *Sidaway v Royal Bethlem Hospital* 1985

However, public opinion on this matter is changing rapidly, and decisions in other countries with similar jurisprudence have taken the patient's perspective, penalising the doctor for not telling the patient enough about the treatment. The UK seems likely to follow suit (Anonymous 1994).

The Medicines Act 1968 clearly allows for doctors to prescribe unlicensed and off-label drugs and therefore this practice is not illegal, i.e. a *criminal* action cannot be brought against a doctor in these circumstances. The most frequent cases brought before the courts relating to end-of-life care involve withholding or withdrawal of treatment and use or misuse of opioids, and not drugs used beyond licence.

Thus, the main risk to doctors when using unlicensed or off-label drugs is whether they are open to a *civil* action for negligence. When using a drug for a licensed indication, the doctor shares liability with the drug manufacturer, but the doctor assumes full liability for the consequences of the drug's actions when it is used off-label or in an unlicensed way. In all cases the standard of care takes precedence over any licensing issues. A civil action can arise when the doctor has a duty of care to a patient, and the duty has been breached and resulted in foreseeable injury to the patient. Although the standard of care expected by a doctor is largely determined by the Bolam principle (i.e. acting in accordance with a reasonable body of medical opinion), there has been a recent addition to this, called the Bolitho modification. This states that, despite a reasonable body of supporting medical opinion, a doctor's actions must still be logical, supportable by evidence and able to withstand cross examination. If these conditions are met, then the doctor will not be found negligent. Furthermore, civil actions are rarely pursued if the damages awarded are likely to be minimal. Damages, which are intended to restore the claimant to the position he or she would have been in but for the negligence, take into account life expectancy and loss of earnings. For a patient who is unwell with a terminal illness, it is likely that any potential damages would be minimal, and this deters potential litigation, even if there may have been a *prima facie* adequate case of negligence.

Is there any research evidence on how doctors in palliative care give information and seek consent from their patients before prescribing? A recent study by Pavis and Wilcock (2001) has shed valuable light on this topic. By means of a postal survey of 182 physicians working in the speciality, which resulted in a 64% response rate, they established that only 2% of units are operating a specific policy regarding prescribing beyond licence: it is limited to trained specialists in 17% of units. Verbal consent was always obtained by only 4% of units, and never by 38%. Regarding written informed consent, 93% of respondents stated that they never sought this. Only 5% always recorded in the patients' case notes when a drug was being used beyond licence and the reasons for this; 50% stated that they never did so. Only 3% always informed other healthcare professionals about such medication; 68% sometimes informed them, whereas 21% never did so.

The survey asked palliative medicine specialists to identify which drugs and routes they used beyond licence. The most common examples offered included ketamine, octreotide, ketorolac, midazolam, gabapentin, amitriptyline, glycopyrrolate, methadone, dexamethasone and hyoscine hydrobromide. These are among the drugs most commonly used in palliative care, particularly in very sick patients near the end of life, and the potential for ADRs and interactions arising is presumably high. There are unfortunately no data, as with the studies in paediatrics discussed above, on the true picture of the consequences of such prescribing.

What are the rights and responsibilities of patients and carers?

Reference has been made above to the right of the patient to receive information, in order to reach a decision about giving (or implying) consent to a medical intervention. The UK Patient's Charter, and forthcoming European legislation, will increase the rights of the individual, sometimes over the medical freedom of the clinician.

How can a patient convey his wishes to the doctor? The conscious patient may signal consent expressly by words or by gesture; written (signed) consent is not a legal requirement and, anyway, may not indicate true consent. However, the patient should still be asked to agree to any specific interventions proposed. Moreover, the patient may legitimately withdraw consent at any time before or during treatment, and such refusal or withdrawal overrides any earlier consent. In the face of refusal, doctors may seek to persuade the patient to change his or her mind, but undue pressure must not be exerted: consent obtained under duress is invalid (Anonymous 1997).

In an unconscious patient, assessment of capacity is not possible and the patient's specific wishes will probably be unknown. In these circumstances, a relative's consent to treatment on behalf of an unconscious or incompetent adult has no legal standing. Nevertheless, consulting relatives and involving them in the decision-making is considered good clinical practice. This is particularly relevant to palliative care, where family-based decision-making is actively encouraged from the earliest contact, and can proceed naturally to carer-only involvement when a patient slips into delirium or unconsciousness. Whatever the relative's wishes, the doctor can treat the unconscious patient only according to his or her 'best interests'.

Along with increasing rights should go greater responsibilities. Thus, it is important for members of the public, whether they are current or potential patients, to become better acquainted and indeed educated about modern medications and routes of delivery. They can only do this, however, if the information is made available to them, in ways that they can readily access and in a language that they can understand. Patient information leaflets (PILs) are now legally bound to be inserted into all dispensed patient packs (Raynor & Britten 2001). These are legally required to give the key facts about indications, expected side effects and contraindications. As such, they may frighten many patients and unduly deter them from complying with the prescribed medication. If the prescription is for an off-label or unlicensed use, the risk of inducing fear and precipitating withdrawal from therapy may be even greater.

Patients are increasingly turning to new technologies for medical information, including television, CD-ROMs and the internet. There are great opportunities for medicine to improve the access to, and quality of, these sources of information. One project that is attempting to empower patients, and to increase their own participation in learning about their condition and its treatments, is PIES (Ahmedzai *et al.* 2001). This stands for personalised information, education and support for cancer patients, and is an internet and videophone-based approach to making such information more accessible. As well as presenting patients with information that is matched to their requirements, PIES encourages patients (and carers) to learn how to use this information more effectively. PIES is still in development and is currently being tested in a regional cancer network around Sheffield.

What are the duties and contributions of pharmacists?

The pharmaceutical profession has a potentially major role to play in the regulation and improvement of prescribing beyond product licences. First, pharmacists are more aware, by virtue of their training and the nature of their posts, of the legislation regarding drug prescribing and dispensing. They have a duty to point out if a clinician appears to have made an error in a prescription, such that the result would take the drug out of the conditions of its licence. This is most likely to occur if the doctor writes a dose that is inordinately high (or low), or if an unusual and potentially ineffective or dangerous route is prescribed. In palliative care (as, indeed, in paediatrics and other areas of medicine, as we have seen above) these situations may arise frequently. It would be intolerable if a pharmacist had to telephone a doctor in palliative medicine every time he or she issued such a prescription, for situations that are clearly regarded by peers and the literature as acceptable practice. A pharmacist should learn which drugs are frequently used in off-label or unlicensed ways, and thus will come to question only the more glaring examples, in which a real error may have been made.

The pharmacist also has a duty of care to the patients, to provide information and clarify information that they may have received from other sources. This is especially relevant to community pharmacists, who are easily contacted by patients and carers in an environment that allows for better communication than a busy hospital setting. Relatively few specialist palliative care units have clinical pharmacists, but, where these are employed or visit from a local hospital or community pharmacy, they may bring substantial benefit to the service.

Pharmacists also have a duty to make available drugs that may be used at short notice in the community, for the care of terminally ill patients who wish to remain at home. Such patients may need very high doses of analgesics, antiemetics and sedatives for subcutaneous infusion, and drugs such as anti-muscarinics for the relief of terminal respiratory airways noise (so-called 'death rattle'). Most of these are off-label, and some are unlicensed uses. A recent survey of all UK regional pharmacy bodies has revealed the lack of standardisation regarding which drugs are made available for out-of-hours use in palliative care (C Hardman and SH Ahmedzai, unpublished data).

Out of 106 local pharmaceutical committees (LPCs) that were surveyed, 81 (76%) responded. When asked if they had a local system 'whereby a named pharmacy or pharmacies will guarantee to stock a supply of commonly prescribed drugs for palliative care', only 46% of respondents were able to reply positively. A further 16% indicated that an 'informal arrangement' was in place, and 10% were considering or planning such an arrangement. Of the LPCs that had pharmacies that guaranteed to stock palliative care drugs, 81% also indicated that they provided an out-of-hours service. In the local schemes, the number of pharmacies that participated ranged from 1 to 6. Only 28% indicated that there was health authority funding for this local service. Notably, out of the 20 drugs and dose forms that these pharmacies cumulatively provided for palliative care, only two were for use within a product licence.

What is the role of palliative care nursing?

Palliative care is a speciality in which nursing has a very important place. This is partly because a large component of palliative care is directed towards giving physical comfort, using strategies not dependent on drug prescribing but rather on traditional nursing procedures. It is also because of the emphasis placed on psychological care, which trained nurses are well placed to offer. The multidisciplinary team working, which is an implicit aspect of palliative care services, also ensures that nurses play a significant role in influencing clinical decision-making.

At the bedside, the nurse may become the patient's closest confidant(e) and so may reach the best understanding of the patient's perception of his or her problems, and how far they will go to have these relieved. In the discussion of whether to initiate an off-label or unlicensed medication, therefore, nurses may act as the patients' advocates, but are potentially also important allies of physicians in communicating with, and obtaining consent from, patients. The final responsibility for taking consent and prescribing is of course with the doctor, but often in palliative care this function is only made feasible and safer by close working with a nursing team.

Nurses are often responsible for handing out published clinical information, and may increasingly be involved in assisting the patient to use newer information and communication technologies such as the internet, particularly in the future through projects such as PIES. After drugs have been prescribed, it is often the nurse who is closest to the patient and who obtains feedback on its effectiveness and the occurrence of side effects.

A new role for nursing in the UK is the imminent growth of nurse prescribing. After successful piloting of the scheme from 1994, community nurse prescribing is planned to be introduced in England. This is based on the recommendations of the 1989 Crown Report on improving nursing care in the community. Nurses working in community NHS trusts or as practice nurses, and who hold the Health Visitor or District Nurse qualifications (or equivalents), and who have completed an approved training course are entitled to prescribe from a limited *Nurse Prescribers' Formulary* (NPF). Nurse prescribing was intended to be fully implemented in 2001, when around 26,000 nurses will be qualified to prescribe: however, this is now likely to be delayed. The NPF consists of a list of drugs, dressings and appliances published as an appendix of the *British National Formulary*. Most of the products can be purchased from pharmacies, although a few are prescription-only medicines.

Nurse prescribing is intended to be substitute, not additional, prescribing because it will mainly involve those products historically prescribed by GPs at the request of nurses. This aims to legitimise existing practice, resulting in more effective patient care and better use of GP, nurse and patient time. As a result, part of GPs' unified budgets has been allocated to nurse prescribing. To aid newly qualified nurse prescribers in England, the National Prescribing Centre is currently publishing a series of educational support materials. Seven *Prescribing Nurse Bulletins* will be sent to all qualified nurse prescribers. One of these is on pain control, and covers the use of paracetamol and aspirin. The bulletins are also available to browse or download from the internet and the NHSNet (http://www.npc.co.uk). At present it is too early to say to what extent nurse prescribing will impact on palliative care practice. The latest recommendations seem to include the prescription of drugs off-label or for unlicensed use.

How can palliative medicine develop a long-term plan for rationalising prescribing beyond licence?

It will be clear from the preceding discussion that prescribing drugs in off-label or unlicensed situations is widespread and almost inevitable in most areas of medicine. In palliative medicine, it is particularly common, and the reasons that are usually stated for this can be summarised as follows:

- Palliative medicine is a relatively new speciality and the evidence base for its interventions is still underdeveloped; accordingly, many of its medication regimens have not been formally researched and are without an appropriate licence.
- As a result of the sensitivities surrounding the care of people near the end of life, conducting conventional research, especially randomised clinical trials (RCTs), in order to establish the case for new licences is very problematic.
- Communication between patients and palliative medicine specialists is regarded to be relatively good, owing to emphasis placed on this issue in the doctors' training – this protects the patients from harm by ensuring their information and consent.

Let us examine these arguments in detail. First, there is the undisputed observation that the evidence for many palliative medicine interventions is lacking, especially from RCTs. Should this be a perpetual excuse for practising medical interventions that have little or no basis in science? While RCT evidence is being gathered, what can the speciality do to ensure more scientifically sound and more consistent prescribing? At least three measures or actions could be implemented. The first is a development from the Science Committee of the Association for Palliative Medicine, which has started to document and review the evidence base of the discipline's treatments, using a pragmatic approach that incorporates both RCTs and less strictly controlled studies (Bennett & Ahmedzai 2000). The Science Committee's task groups are tackling specific clinical questions and producing guidelines, and also recommendations for further research (Mannix *et al.* 2000). These will highlight the areas where regimens are currently beyond product licences and will indicate where special caution should be exercised.

Another step would be to conduct multicentre prospective data-gathering exercises, such as those published by Conroy *et al.* (2000). These would build on the single-centre work of Atkinson and Kirkham (1999) and Todd and Davies (1999), to document how many drugs are used, and in what ways, in different clinical settings and patient populations. As palliative care expands to incorporate more diagnostic groups, this could potentially increase the scope for it to prescribe off-label or in an unlicensed way – this too needs to be documented as it happens.

A third initiative would be the establishment of special reporting mechanisms for consistent and speedy feedback on ADRs as well as efficacy. The model of the PRMC, described above by Clarkson *et al.* (2000), could be replicated in palliative care. This could have other benefits in terms of collaborative data collection, not only for the purposes of clarifying off-label and unlicensed prescribing and their consequences.

Recently, the UK government has allowed restricted research into the potential benefits of cannabis and its derivatives. Synthetic derivatives of cannabis such as nabilone have been used in the UK since the 1980s, initially within a licence as an antiemetic for cancer chemotherapy (Ahmedzai *et al.* 1983), but increasingly for a variety of indications such as pain, dyspnoea and cancer-related anorexia (Atkinson & Kirkham 1999; Campbell *et al.* 2001). With such a topical and socially sensitive subject as cannabis, it is crucial that there should be very close monitoring of it and its derivatives in all clinical applications, either within clinical trials or in routine off-label or unlicensed usage. A national centre for receiving and cataloguing ADRs arising from palliative care prescribing would be an important step towards ensuring that it becomes safer and more accountable – scientifically, legally and socially.

What of the defence that medications used in palliative care have been originally researched elsewhere, usually in non-cancer populations? This has led to many of the drugs then being used off-label, i.e. for roughly the same indications and with the same formulations, but being applied in a different diagnostic group and perhaps with a different dose range or route of administration. This could itself be regarded as acceptable and, if there were consensus among peers in palliative medicine about dose range, scheduling, route, etc., then that could come to be thoroughly defensible practice. In reality, many of the drugs used for pain and symptom control in palliative care of cancer patients do not have licences that are restricted to non-cancer patients, but rather to a clinical indication, e.g. neuropathy. There is no *prima facie* reason to suspect that neuropathic pain in a cancer patient is very much different from that in a patient with chronic disc prolapse or post-herpetic neuralgia. (The reverse may well be true, however: namely that some pains caused by cancer, e.g. raised intracranial pressure from cerebral metastases, or brachial plexus syndrome caused by an expanding small cell lung cancer in the apex of the thorax, have specific anti-cancer treatments which are probably *not* transferable to non-cancer patients – high-dose dexamethasone, radiation therapy or chemotherapy, respectively, in these examples.)

What palliative medicine therefore needs is the documentation of all such situations where drugs that were originally developed and licensed for use in specific non-cancer scenarios are now routinely used in cancer patients. If consensus were then found on the main administration parameters (reasonable dose range, safe route, etc.) by a representative group of palliative medicine practitioners, backed up by published evidence, this list of 'approved off-label' medications could be made available for reference. In this way, blatant deviations in terms of dosing or untried alterations in formulation could be identified as unapproved, and potentially indefensible, practice. Frankly unlicensed prescriptions, such as 'one-off' re-formulations or chemicals used as drugs, would still need to be visible as such, and the prescribers should be aware of their potentially indefensible status.

Second, it is often claimed that it is difficult, as well as ethically risky, to conduct research such as RCTs in terminally ill patients. Several counter-arguments can be used against this position. First, there are other similar areas in which there is a high mortality rate, in which RCTs and other forms of rigorous research are conducted: phase 1 and phase 2 trials in oncology are one example, studies in intensive care units another. Second, RCTs are not the only method of gaining scientific insight into drug prescribing. Well-designed prospective surveys, as described above, can add to the evidence base, if they are large enough and representative. Retrospective audits are not usually helpful here, apart from checking if agreed procedures have been carried out in a specific setting. Clearly, a major barrier to conducting any form of clinical research in this area, apart from the ethical ones, is funding. It is unlikely that the pharmaceutical industry will support trials into answering these questions, for the same economic reasons that they do not pursue new product licences or extensions of existing ones. However, industry as well as scientific research councils and NHS research sources should be systematically lobbied so that more funding comes to palliative medicine research.

The third argument or justification for off-label and unlicensed prescribing is that, in palliative medicine, the interests of the patients when it comes to prescribing decisions are well protected. In 2001, this could seem patronising, because it is not based on a large body of evidence but a reflective view from palliative care itself; even if it may be largely true, it still needs to be documented. It has been shown that nurses in a hospice unit were unlikely to agree with their patients' own ratings of how far they would go in terms of investigations and treatments (Meystre *et al.* 1997). No rigorous studies have been published in which the communication capabilities – and advocacy role – of palliative care physicians have been formally tested in the context of patients' wishes for different types of medication. This is not, of course, to suggest that palliative care positively seeks to misrepresent patient's wishes and fails to inform them and take their feedback. Rather, it emphasises that palliative care could actually set a lead for other specialities, which receive less training in communication skills, on how to achieve good collaboration between patients and professionals in medical decision-making.

Next steps for palliative medicine to take responsibility for prescribing beyond label

From an organisational perspective, the risks presented by staff (doctors, nurses and pharmacists) in using drugs beyond licence are best managed through a clinical governance culture. Clinical governance is now affecting UK palliative care units operating not only within the NHS, but also the large number of services that are 'independent' – usually supported by local or national charities. Rather than restricting their activities, all organisations should empower staff to educate themselves and take responsibility for their actions within a clinical effectiveness framework. This emphasises the need to have in place mechanisms to inform, change and monitor clinical practice. Clinical organisations could also learn from the airline industry where errors are rigorously sought out, but are viewed as system errors rather than person errors. This requires organisations to examine clinical errors with a view to establishing procedures that reduce the chance of that error being repeated. Clinical governance should be viewed as a process for creating improved clinical outcomes and not used as a barrier to informed and risk managed practice.

The Association for Palliative Medicine, which is the official body representing the professional interests of UK specialists in this discipline, also has an important role in this area. It has acknowledged the responsibility of identifying the best practice with respect to prescribing beyond licence, and is taking steps to clarify the way forward. A conference was organised by the Science Committee of the APM in May 2001, in which the medical, legal and pharmacy views were presented and discussed. Arising from this meeting, the APM Science Committee is now considering a series of further actions. These will include joint meetings with other disciplines which face similar issues, such as pain specialists.

Most importantly, a scheme is urgently needed to classify beyond licence prescribing into: those drugs and indications that are considered off-label but are evidence based, safe and fully justifiable; those that are off-label or unlicensed but are supported by some evidence; and those that are unlicensed and unsupported by any evidence. Recommendations are required about the type of information and consent procedures that will be appropriate for each class of medication. Table 6.3 gives a proposed framework for such a scheme. Even if this method is found acceptable to the profession, much work lies ahead to fill in the huge empty database it will open up. This is clearly a long-term task for palliative medicine and its related professional disciplines.

Note that the proposed schema provides both a system for classifying the legal and scientific basis of the prescription, and also the degree of consent required.

Table 6.3 Proposed classification for prescriptions of medication used in palliative care

	Covered by licence / Good literature / Rational	Not licensed / Good literature / Rational	Not licensed / Poor literature / Rational	Not licensed / No literature / Speculative
Characteristic of medication				
Indication				
Diagnosis				
Route				
Formulation				
Dose				
Scheduling				
Safety and approval	Safe / Approved for all	Intermediate safety / Approved for all	Intermediate safety / Approved for specialists	Potentially unsafe / Not approved
Type of consent required	No specific consent needed	Verbal consent suggested	Verbal (written) consent recommended	Written informed consent required

In order to use this schema, each prescription should be assessed by placing a tick for each row describing characteristics of the regimen (indication, route, dose, etc.), within the column that has the best fit with regard to the existing licence, literature base and justification. A 'rational' use is, for example, the use of hyoscine hydrobromide to reduce discharge from a fistula. A 'speculative' use is, for example, the use of prednisolone to reduce mucus secretions from an oesophageal carcinoma (both examples taken from Atkinson & Kirkham 1999). If all ticks are in the left-hand column, the prescription is fully covered by an existing licence; no specific consent is required. If at least one tick is in the right-hand column, there is little justification for the prescription; written informed consent must be sought as in a clinical trial. Regimens with ticks lying in between have varying degrees of scientific and professional justification; verbal consent should ideally be sought.

Thus, regimens that are fully covered by an existing licence need no specific consent other than the usual discussion between clinician and patient. Regimens with one or more characteristics in the right-hand column should indicate the need for obtaining formal written informed consent, as if the patient were entering a clinical trial. For situations in between, it is advisable that at least verbal consent is sought.

What kind of information can patients expect to receive from their palliative care professionals? Clearly, at present, the PILs placed in dispensed packs of drugs are inadequate and may be misleading and frightening for drugs used beyond licence (Raynor & Britten 2001). C Hardman (unpublished communication) has prepared a set of patient information notes, which are designed to cover the off-label and unlicensed uses of drugs commonly used beyond licence in palliative medicine. These have been designed by consultation with clinicians and patient representatives. They are intended to be placed on the internet where clinicians and patients may have direct access, and from where they can be printed out for local use.

All cancer centres and units in the UK are now obliged, according to the National Cancer Plan, to produce a formulary for palliative care drugs and keep this up date. Many palliative care services are responding by designing their own local formularies, whereas others defer to the excellent published *Palliative Care Formulary* (Twycross *et al.* 1998). An advantage of the latter is that it is regularly maintained and kept up to date in an internet version (www.palliativedrugs.org.uk). Both the printed and internet versions of the *Palliative Care Formulary* show what evidence there is for each medication, and also whether or not the recommended use, dose, route, etc. are covered by a licence.

The future of safe and responsible prescribing in palliative medicine depends on the judicious exploitation of all these approaches, which must be both conventional and new technologies, to search for evidence and to disseminate information, to the professionals and members of the public.

References

Ahmedzai HH, Ahmedzai SH, Procter P, Leadbeater M, Emery D (2001). PIES – Personalised Information, Education and Support for cancer patients. Proceedings of 7th European Congress on Palliative Care, Palermo, Sicily. *European Journal of Palliative Care* **154**

Ahmedzai S (1998). Palliation of respiratory symptoms. In Doyle D, Hanks GWC, McDonald N (eds) *Oxford Textbook of Palliative Medicine*. Oxford: Oxford University Press, pp 583–616

Ahmedzai S, Carlyle DL, Calder IT, Moran F (1983). Anti-emetic efficacy and toxicity of nabilone, a synthetic cannabinoid, in lung cancer chemotherapy. *British Journal of Cancer* **48**, 657–663

Anonymous (1994). Talking about drug treatments: who should what to whom? *Drug and Therapeutics Bulletin* **32** (May)

Anonymous (1997). Managing self-harm: the legal issues. *Drug & Therapeutics Bulletin* **35** (June)

Atkinson CV & Kirkham SR (1999). Unlicensed uses for medication in a palliative care unit. *Palliative Medicine* **13**, 145–152

Bashford JNR, Norwood J, Chapman SR (1998). Why are patients prescribed proton pump inhibitors? Retrospective analysis of link between morbidity and prescribing in the General Practice Research Database. *British Medical Journal* **317**, 452–456

Bennett M & Ahmedzai SH (2000). Evidence-based clinical guidelines for palliative care: the work of the APM Science Committee. *Palliative Medicine* **14**, 453–454

Campbell FA, Tramér MR, Carroll D, Reynolds DJM, Moore RA, McQuay HJ (2001). Are cannabinoids an effective and safe treatment option in the management of pain? A qualitative systematic review. *British Medical Journal* **323**, 13–16

Chalumeau M, Tréluyer JM, Salanave B *et al.* (2000). Off label and unlicensed drug use among French office based paediatricians. *Archives of Disease in Childhood* **83**, 502–505

Clark TE, Edom N, Larson J, Lindsey LJ (2001). Thalomid (thalidomide) capsules: a review of the first 18 months of spontaneous postmarketing adverse event surveillance, including off-label prescribing. *Drug Safety* **24**, 87–117

Clarkson A, Ingleby E, Choonara I, Bryan P, Arlett P (2001). A novel scheme for the reporting of adverse drug reactions. *Archives of Disease in Childhood* **84**, 337–339

Conroy S, Choonara I, Impicciatore P *et al.* (2000). Survey of unlicensed and off label drug use in paediatric wards in European countries. *British Medical Journal* **320**, 79–82

Ferner RE (1996). Prescribing licensed medicines for unlicensed indications. *Prescribers' Journal* **36**, 73–78

Gavrilov V, Lifshitz M, Levy J, Gorodischer R (2000). Unlicensed and off-label medication use in a general paediatrics ambulatory hospital unit in Israel. *Israel Medical Association Journal* **2**, 595–597

Lowe-Ponsford F & Baldwin D (2000). Off-label prescribing by psychiatrists. *Psychiatric Bulletin* **24**, 415–417

McIntyre J, Conroy S, Avery A, Corns H, Choonara I (2000). Unlicensed and off label prescribing of drugs in general practice. *Archives of Disease in Childhood* **83**, 498–501

Mannix K, Ahmedzai SH, Anderson H, Bennett M, Lloyd-Williams M, Wilcock A (2000). Using bisphosphonates to control the pain of bone metastases: evidence-based guidelines for palliative care. *Palliative Medicine* **14**, 455–461

Meystre CJN, Burley NMJ, Ahmedzai S (1997). What investigations and procedures do patients in hospices want? Interview based survey of patients and their nurses. *British Medical Journal* **315**, 1202–1203

Pavis H & Wilcock A (2001). Information giving about the use of drugs outside of their license: a survey of palliative medicine specialists in the United Kingdom *British Medical Journal* in press

Penn RG (1979). The state control of medicines: the first 3000 years. *British Journal of Clinical Pharmacology* **8**, 293–305

Raynor DKT & Britten N (2001). Medicine information leaflets fail concordance test. *British Medical Journal* **322**, 1541

Serradell J & Galle B (1993). Prescribing for unlabeled indications. *HMO Practitioner* **7**, 44–47

Todd J & Davies A (1999). Use of unlicensed medication in palliative medicine. *Palliative Medicine* **13**, 446

Turner S, Longworth A, Nunn AJ, Choonara I (1998). Unlicensed and off label drug use in paediatric wards: prospective study. *British Medical Journal* **316**, 343–345

Turner S, Nunn AJ, Fielding K, Choonara I (1999). Adverse drug reactions to unlicensed and off-label drugs on paediatric wards: a prospective study. *Acta Paediatrica* **88**, 965–968

Twycross R, Wilcock A, Thorp S (1998). *Palliative Care Formulary*. Oxford: Radcliffe Medical Press

Table of cases

Bolam v Friern Hospital Management Committee [1957] 1 WLR 582

Sidaway v Royal Bethlem Hospital Governors and others [1985] 1 All ER 6

Useful websites

Medicines Control Agency: http://www.mca.gov.uk/ourwork/ourwork.htm

British National Formulary: http://www.bnf.org/

palliativedrugs.com: http://www.palliativedrugs.com/index.cfm

PART 4

Clinical practice guidelines and medical error

Chapter 7

Appraisal of available guidelines for the management of cancer pain

Teresa Tate

Clinical guidelines, which are systematically developed to assist healthcare workers and patients with decisions about care, have become increasingly common over the past 20 years. Each year has seen an exponential rise in the number of guidelines, so that there are now several hundred available, mainly relating to the medical specialities. This increase perhaps reflects the recent enthusiasm for using evidence and for the demonstration of uniformity and equity in clinical practice.

The first commentary on the potential of clinical guidelines may be traced back to the fourth century BC, when Plato explored the differences between skills that were grounded in practical expertise and those that were based solely on following instructions or obeying rules. Using the clinician as a model, he propounded an experiment in which doctors would be stripped of their clinical freedom and 'no longer allowed unchecked authority'. They would be required to form themselves into councils to determine a majority view about practice in any given situation. They would then codify the decisions of these councils, which he specified should be composed of both clinical and non-clinical members, and publish them to 'dictate the ways in which the treatment of the sick is practised' (cited in Annas & Waterfield 1995).

Plato recognised that a logical consequence of introducing guidelines was that adherence to them would become expected. Deviation from them would be increasingly condemned, until ultimately it would be necessary to make them legally enforceable. In England and Wales we have not yet reached a situation of compulsory implementation of guidelines. Indeed the National Health Service Executive (NHSE 1998) has stated that guidelines cannot be used to mandate, authorise or outlaw treatment options. However, in other parts of Europe, legal actions have already been initiated following the suggestion that participants in guideline developments have conducted themselves improperly.

Many anxieties are inspired by the escalating introduction of clinical guidelines. In particular, the concerns that they erode and diminish the use of clinical judgement and have the capacity to reduce medical practice to the level of 'cookbook' medicine are not new. Plato specifically defined the principle of medicine as an art as well as a science, which should not be hemmed in by rules and which should allow the patient to be considered as a specific, rather than as an average, individual. These concepts are fundamental to palliative care which emphasises the uniqueness of each patient within his or her family unit and his or her right to autonomy and to individualised treatment. They highlight the difficulty for some palliative care clinicians of accepting the entire concept of rule-driven practice.

Within the past 10 years, several organisations have attempted to define and grade the nature and content of guidelines in order to ensure that they are of high quality and are as appropriate as possible. The NHSE suggests that clinical guidelines should aim to achieve many attributes (Table 7.1). Given the same evidence and using the same methods, another group of developers should be able to come to the same recommendations. The recommendations should be interpreted by different professionals facing the same clinical problem in the same way. The guidelines should have a clearly defined target group of patients and should be reviewed and auditable on a regular basis. Crucially, however, they should also allow exceptions in practice and patient preferences to be identified.

Table 7.1 Implementing clinical practice guidelines: can guidelines be used to improve clinical practice? (NHSE 1998)

Valid	Leading to the results expected of them
Reproducible	Given the same evidence and methods of guideline development, another group of developers will come to the same results
Reliable	Given the same clinical circumstances, different health professionals interpret and apply the guidelines in the same way
Cost-effective	Leading to improvements in health at acceptable costs
Representative	By involving the contribution of key groups and interests in their development
Clinically applicable	Patient populations affected are unambiguously defined
Flexible	By identifying exceptions to recommendation as well as the patient preferences to be used in decision-making
Clear	Unambiguous language is used and readily understood by clinicians and patients
Reviewable	The date and process of review will be stated
Amenable to clinical audit	Should be capable of translation into explicit audit criteria

If all the suggestions of the NHSE are observed and guidelines of high quality can be produced, there is evidence to show that using such guidelines has clinical advantage (Norheim 1999). Guidelines have a considerable impact in reducing variations in practice and in controlling costs by limiting treatment options. They improve outcomes, e.g. the use of a pain algorithm significantly reduced complaints of pain in patients based in the community, compared with a control group. Unfortunately, even after more than 20 years, the quality and thus the value of most clinical guidelines can be considered poor (Cluzeau 2000). Many guidelines, particularly those developed by single speciality organisations, have little wider relevance. There is even some evidence that recommendations produced on the same topic by different groups can be conflicting in their content and thus unreliable and irrelevant. If guidelines are produced without using rigorous criteria for their development, their credibility will continue to be undermined and, possibly more seriously, patients may be put at risk if the recommendations are inaccurate (Grilli *et al*. 2000).

There has been debate about the applicability of guidelines. It has been suggested that, if the guidelines are produced by a group of self-selected experts, who are believed to be insulated from the realities of clinical practice, they are more likely to be valid but are less likely to be implemented (Grimshaw *et al*. 1995). Farmer (1993) wrote 'unless a guideline accurately reflects the routine working practices of most doctors, it will act only as a gold standard to be admired and then ignored'. Plato also commented that if 'guideline creation is not routed in the mental processes of clinicians but in the minds of developers distant from the consultation its value is dismissed'.

In the past few years, several authors have discussed the need to develop a system of critical appraisal of practice guidelines. Several measures have been shown to have important implications for the successful implementation of a guideline. Many of these measures have been brought together in the work of Grilli *et al*. (2000). Their measures are not complete and a process of evolution is required to develop a fully validated assessment tool. They have, however, identified three key components, each confirmed by the work of other agencies, which may be used as a checklist.

- Guidelines should be developed with multiprofessional participation of the speciality physicians, other physicians and healthcare providers, and patients. The balance of disciplines within a guideline development group has considerable influence on the resulting recommendations. The names and professions of each of the committee members should be recorded in the publication.
- The strategy used to identify the primary evidence must incorporate a broad base of sources, including electronic databases, and must be recorded.
- An explicit grading of the evidence is required to support each recommendation.

Four currently available guidelines on the management of cancer pain have been assessed according to these criteria of Grilli:

1. *Morphine in Cancer Pain: Modes of administration* (Expert Working Group of the European Association for Palliative Care 1996).
2. *Guidelines for Managing Cancer Pain in Adults* (National Council for Hospice and Specialist Palliative Care Services: Working Party on Clinical Guidelines in Palliative Care 1998).
3. *Principles of Pain Control and Palliative Care for Adults* (Royal College of Physicians: Working Group of the Ethical Issues in Medicine Committee 2000)
4. *Control of Pain in Patients with Cancer* (Scottish Inter-Collegiate Guidelines Network 2000).

The European Association for Palliative Care (EAPC) and Royal College of Physicians (RCP) Guidelines were developed by uniprofessional groups. There is no evidence of a complete systematic review and no grading of the advice given. The National Council for Hospice and Specialist Palliative Care Services (NCHSPCS) guidelines were evolved by a biprofessional group, although the professions of the working group members are not clearly stated in the document. There was no review or grading of the evidence. The Scottish Inter-Collegiate Guidelines Network (SIGN) guidelines were developed by a multiprofessional group, basing its searches on systematic review, meta-analyses and randomised controlled trials. All the recommendations have been graded. It is important to note that all these guidelines are mainly focused on the treatment of pain and contain only brief recommendations stressing the importance of assessment and diagnosis of the specific cause of each pain suffered by the cancer patient.

The considerable importance of developing very accurate guidelines is demonstrated by a recent survey by the NCHSPCS (Finlay *et al.* 2000a). This reviewed all locally available guidelines on the management of pain that are currently in use by specialist palliative care services in England and Wales. The review identified inconsistencies and errors in many parts of the documents submitted, even those that claimed to be directly based on the Council's own guidelines. There were examples of incorrectly spelled drugs, wrongly recommended doses, drugs generally considered inappropriate for use in the management of cancer pain, and a mix of advice on a suitable starting dose of morphine, the gold standard drug. These findings are consistent with those of another author who has described the probability that user involvement in the creation of guidelines will increase the likelihood of their local acceptance, but not guarantee their validity (Grimshaw & Russell 1994). Clearly, if this local adaptation is based on a national guideline that has not met a rigorous standard, there is even more risk of perpetuating errors.

In a clinical environment where physicians are constantly bombarded with more information, directly or indirectly relevant to their practice, than can be easily absorbed, a degree of order is required. The use of guidelines is a practical solution, but it is essential to ensure that these guidelines have credibility and acceptability, and that they maintain the balance between the framework of the guideline and the flexibility required to suit the individual patient's situation in an explicit way (Finlay *et al.* 2000b). Guidelines should support and not constrain the action of clinicians. The relevance of this is demonstrated in the USA where physicians may not claim, as a defence to a charge of negligence, that their clinical judgement has been corrupted by the imposition of a practice guideline (*California Reporter* 1986).

An international collaboration named AGREE (Appraisal of Guidelines Research and Evaluation) will bring together many agencies within the European Union in an attempt to establish frameworks for the development and monitoring of clinical guidelines (AGREE Collaboration 2000). The National Institute for Clinical Excellence will adopt this methodology in its guideline programme. Such a framework should ensure that, in the future, guidelines will be internationally applicable and based on a complete spectrum of graded evidence.

References

AGREE Collaboration (2000). Guideline development in Europe: an international comparison. *International Journal of Technology and Assessment of Health Care* **16**, 1036–1046

Annas J & Waterfield R (eds) (1995). *Statesman.* Cambridge: Cambridge University Press, pp xvi–xvii, 60–61

California Reporter (1986). Wickline v. California. *California Reporter* **228**, 661–667

Cluzeau F (2000). AGREE – A generic appraisal instrument for use worldwide. *Guidelines in Practice* **3**, 14

Expert Working Group of the European Association for Palliative Care (1996). Morphine in cancer pain: modes of administration. *British Medical Journal* **312**, 823–826

Farmer A (1993). Medical practice guidelines: lessons from the United States. *British Medical Journal* **307**, 313–317

Finlay IG, Bowdler JM, Tebbit P (2000a). *Are Cancer Pain Guidelines Good Enough?* London: National Council for Hospice and Specialist Palliative Care Services

Finlay IG, Bowdler JM, Tebbit P (2000b). Criteria for adapting national cancer pain guidelines for local use. *Guidelines in Practice* **3**, 32–43

Grilli R, Magrini N, Penna A, Mura G, Liberati A (2000). Practice guidelines developed by specialty societies: the need for a critical app raisal. *The Lancet* **355**, 103–106

Grimshaw J & Russell I (1994). Achieving health gain through clinical guidelines. *Quality in Health Care* **3**, 45–52

Grimshaw J, Eccles M, Russell I (1995). Developing clinically valid practice guidelines. *Journal of Evaluation of Clinical Practice* **1**, 37–48

NHS Executive (1998). Clinical guidelines: Using clinical guidelines to improve patient care within the NHS. In *Guidelines;* vol 5. Berkhamsted, Herts: Medendium Group Publishing Ltd, pp 13–14

Norheim OF (1999). Healthcare rationing – are additional criteria needed for assessing evidence based clinical practice guidelines? *British Medical Journal* **319**, 1426–1429

Scottish Intercollegiate Guidelines Network (2000). *Control of Pain in Patients with Cancer. A national clinical guideline.* Edinburgh: Royal College of Physicians

Working Group of the Ethical Issues in Medicine Committee (2000). Principles of pain control in palliative care for adults. *Journal of the Royal College of Physicians of London* **34**, 350–352

Working Party on Clinical Guidelines in Palliative Care (1998). *Guidelines for Managing Cancer Pain in Adults*, 2nd edn. London: The National Council for Hospice and Specialist Palliative Care Services

Chapter 8

Understanding, minimising and managing clinical error

Mary Brennan and Rob George

Introduction

As practitioners, our duty to deliver best care ought to be our central motivation. Anticipating, monitoring and managing error are essential, but badly performed, parts of this. The purpose of this chapter is to explain and offer practical ways of managing error as part of good clinical practice.

We begin by setting the epidemiological context of errors and continue by highlighting the vulnerability that seems to be a part of medicine and issues specific to palliative medicine. After an outline of theory on the nature of errors and two possible ways in which to view them, we conclude with practical guidelines and a brief discussion on the use of information technology (IT) in the management of prescribing practice.

The general context

Incidence

This chapter is concerned primarily with errors in prescribing for pain control. It would be helpful if we had direct information on such clinical mistakes and their causes. Sadly, specific data are not available. However, we should be able to get a handle on mistakes by looking generally at adverse events as a proxy for the incidence of errors.

In the 1980s a multicentre Harvard study (Leape *et al.* 1991) reviewed more than 30,000 inpatient records in 51 New York State hospitals and reported that 3.7% of hospital admissions were associated with adverse events (defined as injuries caused by medical management that prolonged admission or produced disability at the time of discharge). Further analysis showed that 69% of these injuries were avoidable. From this work it is estimated that more than 100,000 patients die in the USA each year because of clinical error. This is more than the sum of deaths caused by all trauma, suicide, falls and poisonings. A similar study undertaken in Australia in 1995 reported that 16.6% of hospital admissions were associated with adverse events, half of which were thought to have been avoidable (Wilson *et al.* 1995). In these studies, approximately half of the adverse events related to surgery but the remainder were from diagnostic or therapeutic mistakes, about 20% of which were the result of drug treatments.

Although the Harvard study is likely to offer the best-case scenario – strict definitions of adverse events were applied and only those that resulted in injury were captured – both studies give credence to the use of adverse events as a proxy for identifying and investigating error. One thing that can be said is that errors are unacceptably common, but, more importantly, it is said that only about 1 in 10 of errors and near misses is reported.

There are no comparable large-scale studies from UK hospitals in the literature. However, a recent pilot study reviewed more than 1,000 medical records retrospectively in two acute hospitals in Greater London and reported that 10.8% of patients experience adverse events (overall adverse event rate of 11.7% when multiple events are included) (Vincent *et al.* 2001). Once again it was judged that half of these are preventable. These figures support the Chief Medical Officer's assumption that up to 850,000 adverse events might occur in NHS hospitals each year at a cost of over £2bn (Department of Health 2000). This represents a significant burden in terms of both human suffering and finance on our healthcare system.

Looking specifically at studies that address problems with medication, Bates *et al.* (1995) report that 6.5% of patients admitted to hospital have adverse drug events and a further 5.5% have the potential for them. They found that over a quarter of these were the result of errors, implying that more than 3% of hospitalised patients are at risk of harm from avoidable, serious, medication errors. Finally, of the adverse drug events, 1% were fatal, 12% life threatening, 30% serious and 57% deemed significant.

In the management of clinical risk, it is relatively easy to focus on drug errors as fertile ground for improvement: they are common and mainly preventable. Bates *et al.* (1998) also provide evidence that 5% of prescriptions have mistakes; these are remediable. This is illustrated well by an interventional study in a UK renal unit, which introduced electronic prescribing to minimise errors (Nightingale *et al.* 2000). The results were impressive. The problems of transcription errors and illegibility were eliminated and unsafe prescriptions were flagged up and stopped. The impact was to reduce erroneous prescriptions to less than 0.1% using a system that was more acceptable to users than the previous manual one. We return to IT at the end of the chapter.

In summary, drug errors are a substantial and reducible source of clinical risk to patients, so why have we not sorted it out long ago? One possibility is our attitude.

The professional context

At the time of writing, with one or two notable exceptions (microbiology and transfusion medicine) (Williamson *et al.* 1998, 1999; Love *et al.* 2000), a random look at the newspapers confirms beyond a reasonable doubt that there is a pervading climate in medicine that has distorted our perceptions of error and its management. This has led, on the one hand, to conspiracies of silence in the face of chronic incompetence, negligence and systematic failure (one example being 'Bristol') or, on the other, to the pursuit of individuals on the grounds that clinical error is indicative of individual technical weakness or moral turpitude. If only life were that simple (Wu 2000; Berwick 2001). We pick up on this dichotomy later.

One explanation of this type of behaviour may be the apparent lack of personal insight among clinicians when reflecting on their individual practice. This was shown clearly in an international study comparing the attitudes to error and stress of operating theatre staff, intensive care unit (ICU) staff and surgeons, with those of aviation cockpit staff (Sexton *et al.* 2000). They found that, generally, clinical staff do not recognise the effects of fatigue on performance (70% surgeons and 47% anaesthetists versus 26% pilots). But it gets worse. Astonishingly, about a third of ICU staff do not believe that they make mistakes and, of those that do, half find it hard to talk of the mistakes that they acknowledge. In other words, only a sixth have insight into their frailties and are able to speak of them. There was a fragment of reality in that two-thirds of clinical staff in this study felt that errors were managed inappropriately in their hospital and that teamworking was poor. Sadly, although the stereotype of the unaccountable and arrogant doctor finds much support in this piece, surprisingly the nurses studied did not come out a great deal better. Neither group gets anywhere near the aircrews in terms of their awareness of personal frailties or recognition of the value of teamwork in reducing the risks of error.

We do not have data on clinicians in palliative care or pain management and it would be tempting to think that our commitment to teamwork and reflective practice would militate against similar finding. That would be very rash. It is best to assume that we are no better than our surgical and anaesthetic colleagues. However, there are some issues particular to palliative care and pain management that are worth airing.

Some specific issues in pain management and palliative care
External perceptions (colleagues and families)

Here we wish to highlight two issues that may confound the monitoring or accuracy of error reporting in palliative care and pain management. These are the popular perceptions that death is medical failure and that opiates kill (as rife in our colleagues as in the general population). We need, however, to include in this short but important section a cluster of principles to explain how perceptions can distort others' views of good and safe practice and open us to charges of clinical error or even gross malpractice, when no such thing was happening.

False premises and flawed logic

All of our lines of logic start with premises. Necessarily, the conclusions to such processes are only correct if both premise and locution are valid and correct. Let us use some oversimplified but valid examples to illustrate the point.

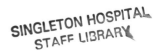

A deduction based on a false premise: death is medical failure

To begin with premises, if one believes that all diseases are actually or potentially curable (*premise 1*), then, logically, a patient faced with the problem of illness will go to any length to find a cure. Similar logic dictates that a physician with the same preconception will never stop trying to cure his or her patients. Under this false premise, our patient and doctor are likely (using correct logic) to conclude that patients die from inadequate or wrong treatments, or medical failure, rather than the natural progression of their illness. The solution to this conclusion is to find the problem or error and not to do it again.

> Statement 1, that patients die from failed, inadequate or wrong treatments, or medical failure, is false.

Let us now build our example with another almost universal premise: that all processes are part of a flow of cause and effect provided that you look hard enough (*premise 2*), which for this argument we take to be correct. This will now dictate the manner in which we draw conclusions – deductions by applying logic alone, or inductions by using evidence to support the logic – and find the cause – there will always be one. Finally, we are taught that, when we find one explanation to account for a cluster of observations, then it is likely to be the correct one, i.e. do not come up with three explanations when one will do. This is known as Ocham's razor (*premise 3*).

> Premise 3, that if there is one explanation for a constellation of events it is likely to be correct, is not always true.

In summary, the premise that patients die of medical failure/error is false and that there is always a single 'culprit' (*premises 2* and *3*) is also wrong. Let us move on to see how else we can go astray using flawed logic.

An induction based on flawed logic: palliative physicians kill their patients with opiates

There is a common inference laid at the door of palliative care that we kill many of our patients with opiates. This is a good example of a false conclusion, which is based principally on flawed logic, but sits on slightly shaky foundations: the shadow of premise 1 and statement 1 (false), premise 2 (true) and Ocham's razor, which may be blunt. Crudely, the argument goes as follows:

> Statement 2: Opiates have the pharmacological potential to kill and have been used to kill. Is there evidence?

In 2000 a British GP, Harold Shipman, was convicted for dispatching scores of his patients with intravenous injections of diamorphine – all the victims were well, all were opiate naïve and exhumed bodies contained opiates. *Premise 2 **plus** the evidence* make the statement true (beyond reasonable doubt!) that he killed with opiates. *Statement 2 is true.* (We use this example as it is very much in the public mind at the time of writing, and as a result, we now have several GPs in our area who will prescribe opiates only under direct advice.)

Statement 3: most patients of palliative care doctors die.

Is there evidence? Look at the records. *Statement 3 is true.*

Statement 4: palliative care doctors give their patients much higher doses of diamorphine than Dr Shipman.

Is there evidence? Drug charts and, what is more, most patients are on opiates at the time of death. *Statement 4 is true.*

It is now a very short step for grieving relatives and colleagues, based on premises 1 and 2, to seek, using Ocham's razor, a single explanation for the timing of a death and to conclude, understandably, but naïvely, that, notwithstanding pain, there is a causal link between any increasing opiate prescriptions and a patient's deteriorating condition.

Observing our management of dying patients repeatedly without explanation makes it is very easy to see, among non-specialists in palliative care, how shaky premises linked by flawed logic lead to a general belief that, because opiates *may* kill, by prescribing them to our dying patients we inevitably hasten their demise.

Remember also that clinicians, like our ICU staff (Sexton *et al.* 2000), who aspire to or believe in their clinical infallibility, may be prey to false premise or flawed logic, such as the example cited. It is a human trait that we prefer if possible to allow 'blame' for perceived, personal failings, such as our patients' deaths, to fall on another to assuage any sense of professional or personal guilt. Under these circumstances it is easy to see how an adverse outcome such as a patient's death during chemotherapy can lead to a search for a specific, tangible alternative that can be deemed causal. Opiates are very handy for that.

Poor communication and education

Without a clear understanding of different indications for medications and others' practice, clinicians are naturally suspicious of colleagues who prescribe medications in unfamiliar or apparently excessive doses. A good example would be steroids: rheumatologists, chest physicians and neurologists use very different schedules for the diseases that present to them. However, it is generally known that the therapeutic approaches to polymyalgia rheumatica, acute asthma and raised intracranial pressure are legitimate in their differences, not least because the intent is to reverse the problem. There is a subtle difference in palliation in that our interventions reduce symptoms by masking rather than reversing the cause. This may make an acute clinician edgy because the clinical marker of curative success has been removed and, in their eyes, the disease has been left unchecked and unmonitored. It is not surprising, therefore, that, in some institutions, palliative care doctors are perceived to overdose their patients when their pain is removed. This view can arise because our experience leads us to escalate doses of effective analgesics quickly in the face of increasing pain, knowing this to be safe. We also feel more comfortable with higher doses of opiate than clinicians with less experience in this setting. Their practice (and consequently their comfort zone) may, for example, be limited to much lower dosing schedules and a failure to distinguish absolute values from dose increments. We need to guard against these problems by careful communication, documentation and tireless education. We cannot expect colleagues to accept our recommendations without clear explanation.

The general messages to take from this section are that what appears to be evidence may not be all that it is cracked up to be and things are not always what they seem. In addition, we ought to understand that we are just as vulnerable to errors similar to those that we have just discussed, e.g. we are wedded to the idea that opiates are safe. We must not forget the other side of the razor: familiarity with opiates and loose views of the double effect may make one vulnerable to reckless or cavalier prescribing. Familiarity with narcotics must never lead to contempt for the power of these drugs or ways in which they can cause problems, e.g. the documented risk of toxicity when neuropathies are present. We now move on to see how this influences the way in which we ought to approach clinical errors.

Some theory

There are two polar views that help us to understand some of the tensions in error management: one is the view that there is such a thing as a perfect world that is messed up by individuals, the other that human fallibility is a given and that systems are the only way to minimise error (Reason 2000).

The 'perfect world'

> This is a person-based approach where failure is seen as a vice and an individual's error as the primary cause of an adverse event.

If we believe that a perfect world can exist, any error must be ascribable to specific failings. As the perfect world is man-made, any failings must ultimately be attributable to an individual. Not only does this view seek to blame individuals but a necessary consequence follows: that the threat of disciplinary action or even litigation promotes a climate of cover-up and deception. It centres on reporting *who* failed rather than *why* the error occurred. This approach uses coercion as compliance, uncouples the institution from the error and exposes the individual.

The 'perfect world' view has a personal focus that seeks to identify and blame the person who has undertaken the task that led to the problem. It can fail to consider whether the procedure was flawed in the first place or indeed whether the individual was adequately trained and competent to undertake those duties. In these circumstances, it is understandable that in such an environment error reporting is seen as a last resort.

Regrettably this approach is the most prevalent in medicine today in spite of the fact that, in comparable services, such as aviation maintenance, there are data that judge 90% of quality lapses as blameless and the result of a systematic error rather than an individual failing (Sexton *et al.* 2000).

The 'flawed world'

> A system-based approach acknowledges that people are frail and, as a consequence, both they and the systems they create are prone to error.

Errors tend to occur in a particular set of circumstances and, if the circumstances recur, the error is likely to be repeated irrespective of the individuals involved. The 'system defence' recognised as a necessity in the flawed world view protects the blameless individual and secures his or her co-operation to facilitate continuous improvement by reporting *what* failed rather than *who* failed. The approach is evolutionary and creates safeguards and barriers by exposing weaknesses that can then be addressed and rectified into increasingly refined protocols and guidelines.

Reporting errors therefore becomes automatic and leads to positive outcomes. These can even be described as 'free lessons' if a disaster waiting to happen is identified and remedied. A contemporary example would be the use of unique labelling, colouring or connectors to prevent the accidental drawing up or delivery of medications by one route that should be given only by another. Recent examples would be the fatal intrathecal delivery of an intravenous cytotoxic agent or the intravenous rather than epidural administration of bupivacaine (Marcain), which has also recently led to a fatality.

This approach creates an environmental focus promoting optimum conditions for a climate of openness in which errors can be valued for the learning opportunities that they provide. Importantly, the fallible world approach must not ignore the potential that a malevolent or incompetent worker exists. By having good error trend reporting and good teamwork, the activities of 'rogues' are more likely to be evident.

Practical application

Promoting balanced systems

So much for the theory: how do we turn it into useful safeguards?

Prepare the environment (latent conditions)

If we examine mishaps we will find that virtually all were 'waiting to happen' and have a causal history extending back in time and through different levels of the system. Mistakes happen because there are underlying weaknesses ('latent conditions') that provoke errors. In general these are environmental and remedial. To mitigate these risks the involvement and support of the whole organisation is needed.

Error prevention requires:

- *Senior management commitment* to provide a good working environment
- *Appropriate staff structures* with clearly defined areas of responsibility and adequate staffing levels
- *Good training* programmes for all staff.

Define 'the system'

To define the system of safety, organisations must translate broad organisational policies into clear, specific and unambiguous guidelines and procedures. At a procedural level one should be aiming for:

- *The least complex way to achieve a task that includes appropriate checking procedures*. Examples are all around us, such as those undertaken to set up blood transfusions, or the pharmacist's check of patients' drug charts for drug interactions.
- *If changes are necessary to complex procedures they should be piloted in a safe environment*. Life-critical processes should be defined in standard operating procedures (SOPs) which are the basis of staff training. As part of a total quality system, there should be regular review of policies, processes and SOPs, as well as a relevant clinical audit programme.
- *There should be an effective error/near-miss reporting system*. By making errors visible the organisation and workplace can become aware of risk systematically. The organisation also needs to remain non-judgemental for proactive risk management to incorporate automatically into routine processes and practice. The achievable counsel of perfection is to use errors to develop better practice to generalise old errors in an effort to imagine potential new ones!

This leads to the concept of 'no blame' reporting: experience in the USA has shown that non-punitive, voluntary, confidential, error-reporting systems provide more useful, detailed information about errors and their causes than mandatory systems. This is not surprising if you consider the motivation for reporting errors in the different systems. In filing a mandatory report, there is a tendency to provide the minimum data possible to meet the requirement as well as to optimise self-protection. A voluntary report motivated by the intention to provide others with information that can help them avoid a similar pitfall is understandably more informative (Barach & Small 2000).

'The Swiss cheese effect': recognise that policies and procedures, like staff, are fallible

Each layer of defence should be intact but in reality there are likely to be holes. Where these are aligned the system, rather than the individual, will allow an error to slip through. This has been described as the 'Swiss cheese effect'. Those readers who have investigated a serious medical error will no doubt recognise the phenomenon and the fact that serious adverse events almost always follow a sequence of mistakes at different stages, undertaken by different individuals involved in a procedure (Williamson *et al.* 1999). Looking at therapeutics, drug error can arise at any point from prescription (56% of drug errors) to administering the wrong medication at the patient's bedside (24% of drug errors). It can also start with a poorly legible script, misinterpretation by a pharmacist, followed by a failure to challenge an anomaly by the nurse administering the medication.

Prepare the people (active conditions)

Mistakes will happen irrespective of all our precautions. These are unsafe acts that arise randomly and can be described as 'active failures'. They are person-based and unpredictable, such as a lapse of concentration or a procedural violation. In general their impact is usually local and short-lived. We should expect these types of error and as far as possible restrain their effect by teamwork, supervision and error-trend review. These tactics will also pick up poor performers and identify the need for re-training.

There is ample evidence from the aviation industry of the value of good teamworking in reducing the error rate (Sexton *et al.* 2000). In our speciality, we use many techniques including clinical supervision and reflective case studies to develop team members and support them in their work. We need to have monitoring systems that provide information such as trend analysis of prescribing practice that will inform our reviews of clinical policies and clinical audit programmes. These suggestions apply to the whole team – no exceptions for senior staff who are less likely to see supervision and reflective practice as a standard part of their normal working pattern.

Extending nurse roles

Our specialist nurses are advisers now, but they are the prescribers of the future. We must set up systems both to support these practitioners and to ensure patient safety. An outline framework would include the development of clinical policies, protocols (including patient group directives) and standardised procedures. Our staff must be well trained and assessed to be competent in their work. By having systems that are robust and open to clinical audit, we will protect patients from rogue practitioners and clinical error, and our staff from unwarranted criticism.

Accommodating exceptions

It is well recognised that in palliative medicine the treatment of many symptoms involves the use of medications prescribed 'off-licence' in terms of the indication for and/or the dose or route of medication prescribed. Our practice abounds with numerous examples, e.g. carbamazepine, licensed for the treatment of trigeminal neuralgia, but not licensed for use in other neuropathic pains. Similarly we may use the non-steroidal anti-inflammatory drug ketorolac by the unlicensed subcutaneous route, often with good effect. Remember that, while the licensing process regulates the pharmaceutical companies and not a doctor's prescribing practice, as the prescribing doctor you carry the burden of the patient's welfare and in the event of adverse reactions you may be called upon to justify your actions. We need to be constantly aware of the balance between risk and benefit of a particular treatment and to operate within agreed protocols with clearly defined boundaries. This is addressed in Chapters 7 and 11. Most importantly, our practice should be logical, reasonable and defensible when viewed by our peers.

Protocols for prescribing 'off-licence' must include, wherever possible, an explanation to the patient (or perhaps the next of kin) that a particular drug is more commonly used for a different indication or by another route, but in our experience it is helpful in managing their symptoms. This is an area where we strive to balance giving our patients information about their treatment against causing unnecessary anxiety.

Skiing 'off piste'

Even with established protocols for prescribing particular drugs 'off-licence', from time to time there are legitimate and unexpected situations where unanticipated combinations, dosages or routes of administration may need detailed consideration. Such exceptional circumstances need lucid analysis, options appraisal and, most importantly, documentation, with a clear chain of authority and responsibility specifying:

- the points of variance
- the process undergone
- authorisation by senior staff member.

In our service we use the algorithm in Figure 8.1 to manage all prescription exceptions.

Rogue practitioners

Sadly we cannot leave this section without mentioning rogue practitioners. These will always be around and are potentially difficult to control (though mercifully rare). Even so, the mere possibility of a rogue practitioner is sufficient justification to oblige services to have systems that define and control exceptions. This will restrain the

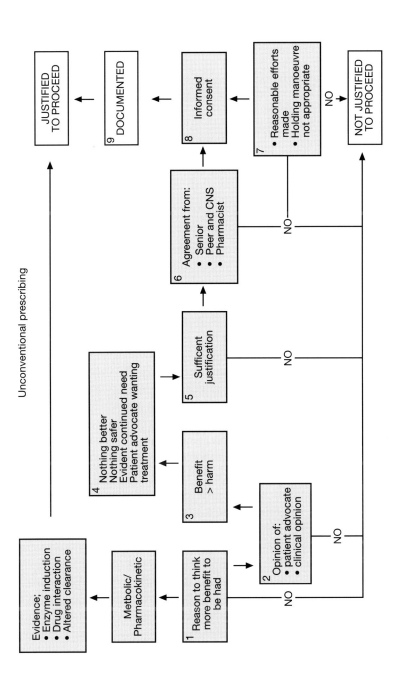

Figure 8.1 The algorithm is used in any situation where there is an unresolved clinical problem and where a drug option is under consideration. We start at point 1 (left-hand side in the middle) and may engage nine stages to justify or forbid our procedure to the next step. The purpose is to ensure that we have been sufficiently rigorous, that there is a chain of authority to consultant level and that we have fulfilled our duty to care by including our patient or the family in deliberations, and that the consenting process has been adequate.

enthusiast and expose the reckless. For those at any level whose character simply does not recognise that they need accountability, no mechanism will hold them. However, an agreed formal protocol will offer an indisputable framework should investigation of an adverse event be necessary.

Specific opportunities to systematise drug prescribing

Prescribing is essentially an algorithmic process and is highly amenable to some form of mechanisation, at least to limit options and specify doses for final clinical decision-making. It therefore cries out for a computerised approach, particularly now that technology is cheap and available.

IT approaches to risk

Computerised systems facilitate audit, research and risk management by providing accurate audit trails and data capture as well as the potential for automatic error reporting. They also allow for developments such as stock control and inventory management.

Electronic prescribing systems

There is evidence that electronic prescribing can reduce clinical error (Nightingale *et al*. 2000). Electronic prescribing systems have advantages over and above manual ones in that they are consistent, accurate and generally reliable. Unlike many doctors' handwriting they are invariably legible. They can be engineered to include safeguards which flag up potential problems that may arise as a result of drug interactions, or as a result of patient-specific characteristics (severe allergy or impaired renal function, etc.). Finally, the system can identify transcription errors or duplication of drugs from the same class.

With refinement and system developments parameters can be established:

- *To offer dose ranges and alarm flags* set for dosing outside ranges in terms either of absolute values or of increments.
- *To recognise errors of omission, and issue reminders* for necessary combinations such as laxatives with opioid prescriptions.
- *To issue minor warnings* that allow a prescription to proceed only after an acknowledgement by the prescriber that he or she is aware of the warning.
- *Major warnings* that cannot be ignored and may require a password to proceed with the prescription (implying that senior staff can take responsibility for a higher risk level) or the reason for variance to be recorded to override a warning.

However, there are downsides. Some computerised prescribing systems have been criticised because they provide too much data, creating confusion, and too much choice. Furthermore these systems rely on significant IT resources, are time-consuming to design, test and implement, and will require ongoing technical support and robust hardware. Packages are increasingly available off the shelf to aid electronic prescribing, but nevertheless a database will only be as good as the data entered. Staff need to be co-operative, competent and committed. Nevertheless, we believe this to be the way forward.

Conclusions

We cannot eliminate all errors, but we have abundant opportunities to minimise them. The lamentable thing in medicine is that we are still failing at the first hurdle, namely our recognition that doctors are as vulnerable to error as anyone. We must not foster the idea that infallibility is achieved along with the status of a senior doctor.

Many, if not most, of our clinical errors are avoidable with simple but necessary measures. We are not good at going back to first principles to find the root causes of errors. We need to learn to examine system weaknesses rather than focus on individuals' errors. The recurring error of intrathecal administration of vincristine is a prime example (Berwick 2001). It has been suggested that chemotherapy protocols should be amended to administer intrathecal methotrexate and intravenous vincristine on separate days, thereby removing the possibility of mixing up the routes of administration or incompatibility of intravenous and intrathecal locking devices. These are not earth-shattering changes in practice or an illegitimate violation of clinical autonomy; they are common sense. Why are we incapable of doing such simple things?

If we recognise that errors always have a context, we will be receptive to the opportunities that a good and effective error reporting system offers to improve our services. This will foster the development of an active learning organisation as opposed to a passive, reactive one. Safety measures need to be engineered into every layer of our organisations. Some defences are low-tech: the development of clinical policies translated into clear standard procedures that are as simple as possible to fulfil the task. A classic example is the procedure to check the administration of controlled drugs. Others will be high-tech, such as the appropriate use of new technologies (computer hierarchies and password-protected activities). Even so, in many aspects safe practice in medicine is still reliant on people. Staff require clarity in defining their roles, responsibilities and accountability as well as robust support systems including appropriate high-quality training. We must ensure that we foster an environment that encourages multidisciplinary teamwork, openness and confidence to challenge unusual circumstances if we are to minimise and manage clinical error.

References

Barach P & Small SD (2000). Reporting and preventing medical mishaps: lessons from non-medical near miss reporting systems. *British Medical Journal* **320**, 759–763

Bates DW, Cullen DJ, Laird N *et al.* (1995). Incidence of adverse drug events and potential adverse drug events: implications for prevention. *Journal of the American Medical Association* **274**, 29–34

Bates DW, Leape LL, Cullen DJ *et al.* (1998). Effect of computerized physician order entry and a team intervention on prevention of serious medication errors. *Journal of the American Medical Association* **280**, 1311–1316

Berwick DM (2001). Not again! *British Medical Journal* **322**, 247–248

Department of Health (2000). *An Organisation with a Memory: Report of an expert group on learning from adverse events in the NHS.* London: Department of Health

Leape LL, Brennan TA, Laird N *et al.* (1991). The nature of adverse events in hospitalised patients: results of the Harvard medical practice study. *New England Journal of Medicine* **324**, 377–384

Love EM, Williamson LM, Cohen H *et al.* (2000). *Serious Hazards of Transfusion Report 1998/1999*

Nightingale PG, Adu D, Richards NT, Peters M (2000). Implementation of rules based computerised bedside prescribing and administration: intervention study. *British Medical Journal* **320**, 750–753

Reason J (2000). Human error: models and management. *British Medical Journal* **320**, 768–770

Sexton JB, Thomas EJ, Helmreich RL (2000). Error, stress and teamwork in medicine and aviation: cross sectional surveys. *British Medical Journal* **320**, 745–749

Vincent C, Neale G, Woloshynowych M (2001). Adverse events in British hospitals: preliminary retrospective record review. *British Medical Journal* **322**, 517–519

Williamson LM, Lowe S, Love E *et al.* (1998). *Serious Hazards of Transfusion Report*

Williamson LM, Lowe S, Love E *et al.* (1999). *Serious Hazards of Transfusion Report 1997/1998*

Wilson RM, Runciman WB, Gibberd RW, Harrison B, Newby L, Hamilton JD (1995). Australian paper. *Medical Journal of Australia* **163**, 458–471

Wu AW (2000). Medical error: the second victim. *British Medical Journal* **320**, 726–727

PART 5

The organisation of clinical services and the delivery of care

Clinical governance and the management of cancer pain: implications and imperatives for the organisation of cancer pain services

Anne Naysmith

Clinical governance has been a priority for all healthcare services in the UK since the publication of *A First Class Service: Quality in the new NHS* (Department of Health 1998). The fundamental concepts of clinical governance are clear: systematic processes in every organisation must maintain high standards of care and minimise clinical risk; the environment must encourage continuous improvement in service quality; and health care should be patient centred with users involved in assessing how well it meets their needs.

Clinical governance is important in cancer pain management, but there are particular difficulties in implementing systematic evaluation in this care setting. Effective governance requires an adequate evidence base on which to define good practice, but this is largely lacking. There are several reasons for this.

Patients with cancer pain are a heterogeneous group. The pain may be of several types – nociceptive, incident and neuropathic are probably the most common – and may arise from the underlying cancer, the effects of previous treatment or an unrelated co-morbid condition. Patients with pain caused by progressive cancer, numerically the largest group, are often in an unstable clinical state. Randomised controlled trials in this group of patients have therefore been difficult to perform. Many studies report on small numbers of patients. The strength of the evidence is therefore poor.

There are many randomised controlled trials in patients with pain from benign conditions, or who experience pain during the early stages of cancer. It is not possible to be certain that the results of trials performed on patients with early disease, or with pain from conditions other than progressive cancer, can be generalised to patients with advanced disease, but in most situations this is the only evidence available.

Deriving valid guidelines from such a limited evidence base is difficult. If a guideline is to be implemented successfully, it needs to be locally owned. Many clinicians therefore prefer to develop treatment protocols locally, rather than use national or international ones which take no account of local needs or organisational structures. However, few local organisations have the necessary skills to develop valid guidelines, particularly from such a limited evidence base (Finlay *et al.* 2000).

It is important that guidelines are developed at a national level in accordance with the available evidence and with wide consensus. Such guidelines need to be widely disseminated, to generalist settings as well as to those that include the management of cancer pain as specialist practice. Resources need to be made available to update such guidelines regularly.

Cancer pain should be managed by a multidisciplinary team, which is to some extent assembled uniquely around each patient. The team will include both the primary care team looking after the patient at home and the specialists in secondary care managing the anti-tumour treatment. Members of the team need to have the necessary training and experience in the management of cancer pain. This often means involving specialists in palliative care. Currently, specialist palliative care teams usually work in an advisory capacity in the UK. They rarely have the resources to provide access to specialist help at all stages of the cancer pathway, in all patient care settings and at all times. Continuity of care is often difficult to maintain across the boundaries between institutions, and between secondary and primary care. If high-quality cancer pain management is to be delivered, the availability of pain management skills must be an integral part of the patient pathway from the diagnosis of cancer onwards. Specialist teams must be available in all settings to offer advice and training to the primary carers, and must be able to take over the care of those with complex and highly demanding ongoing pain problems. This has clear resource implications in terms of the need for suitable doctors, nurses and other professionals. We lack trained specialists in each discipline in sufficient numbers. Most services are available only during limited hours. Although current guidelines for cancer management in the UK state that specialist palliative care advice should be continuously available, 24 hours a day and every day of the week, meeting that standard would require a major expansion in staffing numbers. It is not clear that staff with the necessary specialist skills could be recruited at present, even if there were no financial constraints. Current resources for education may not be adequate to give every member of such a team the necessary training, experience and supervision. As one of the main tasks of the core specialist team is to act as a resource for those caring for patients, most in a non-specialist setting, the lack of sufficient trained professionals in specialist teams also impacts on the skills and knowledge of those working in oncology, primary care and other settings in which patients with cancer pain are managed. It is important that there is continued investment in the training and recruitment of specialist staff, as well as in the training of staff from other specialities. Skills in cancer pain management need to be integral to all hospital and community services for cancer patients, including primary care. The extension of nurse prescribing to include the titration of drug doses in cancer pain management should help to streamline the care process.

There must also be commitment to equity of access to specialist advice and skills. This means that these skills must be uniformly distributed across care settings.

Current evidence suggests that there may be barriers for some patients in accessing specialist services. Groups under-represented in inpatient specialist palliative care include ethnic minorities, those with significant psychiatric illness, such as psychotic illnesses and alcohol abuse (Working Party for the National Council for Hospice and Specialist Palliative Care Services 1995, 2000), and very elderly people. There is no evidence to suggest that these groups are receiving their pain management in other settings. It is imperative that we deliver high-quality cancer pain management purely on the basis of patient need. Services must be designed such that language, cultural or religious beliefs, age or being outside mainstream services does not constitute a barrier.

The most direct measure of successful health care is a valid indicator of good outcome. Such indicators are difficult to derive, particularly in chronic diseases associated with progressive deterioration in overall health and eventual death. Process measures are often used as a practical substitute, particularly if, in a research context, the process being measured can be shown to be associated strongly with the desired outcome. However, in cancer pain management, there is a dearth of good measures of either process or outcome (Hearn & Higginson 1997). We lack good measures of pain that can be uniformly applied. If the patient is capable of assessing his or her own pain repeatedly, using a reproducible scale, then this gives valid information about responses to treatment. Unfortunately, patients often find such assessments too demanding to undertake repeatedly. This becomes more and more the case as the cancer advances, although this is also when pain is likely to be an increasing problem. Proxy measures, supplied by either a professional or a relative or carer, often have to be substituted, particularly as patients become more ill. Proxy measures, particularly from family members, do not correlate well with the patient's own reported pain (Higginson *et al.* 1994). This makes it particularly difficult to compare outcomes either between different clinical settings or across time periods.

Nevertheless, an essential part of clinical governance is the use of audit to measure outcomes against an agreed standard. Outside specialist palliative care services, performance indicators have tended to focus on outcomes such as remission and survival, or process measures such as radical versus palliative radiotherapy. Audit of outcomes such as pain control has been particularly lacking in primary care settings. In cancer pain management, clinical audit has to be carried out across professional and institutional boundaries and to measure achievement against goals, which are agreed with patients and families. This is not part of current practice, and it is difficult to see how it could be performed in the UK with the current resources. Routinely collected data tend to focus on activity, e.g. staff contacts with patients or inpatient stays, rather than on outcome, and does not allow the patient's pathway to be followed across the interfaces between institutional settings, or the contributions of different professions to be integrated. The development of the 'Electronic Health Record' should make this task easier.

Agreeing goals with patients and their families is particularly important in cancer pain management. Families often over-estimate the degree of physical pain that the patient is experiencing. Patients are, however, often reluctant to acknowledge their pain, or to take prescribed analgesia, even when they find that it does relieve their pain. There are probably a number of reasons for the difficulty that patients have in complying with analgesic regimens, and different patients will have different priorities. Success rates might improve if those treating cancer pain took note of the experience gained in managing other chronic diseases, such as asthma. In these, self-management plans have not been as successful as hoped because they did not take into account the patient's own view of his or her illness and psychological needs, trying instead to impose a purely medical model on the experience of being asthmatic. Cancer pain sufferers also experience pain as a metaphor for the advance of their illness and the closeness of death, so that pain comes to be feared out of proportion to its actual severity. Like people with asthma, patients with cancer do not want to hear that their pain is incurable and life-long and needs constant medication. Most continue to hope for a remission from it, either as a result of anti-tumour treatment or simply spontaneously, and try to limit the amount of analgesia that they take. Success rates are likely to improve if health professionals acknowledge the validity of patients' feelings, and try to negotiate agreed goals and a common plan, with which the patient is then more likely to comply.

Even when clinical audit is performed, the outcomes do not always lead to the necessary changes being implemented, either because of the degree of institutional change required or because the necessary resources cannot be identified. Future service development needs to incorporate the need for regular audit in the resource allocation. Nationally agreed audit tools would facilitate comparison between services and settings.

Conclusions

- To improve the evidence base, good randomised controlled trials should be carried out in patients with cancer pain, including those with advanced disease.
- To improve pain management, specialist teams with the right membership, who have had the right training, are in the right place and are available all of the time must be available.
- Training is crucial to the skills of all the members of the care team, particularly those who are not specialists in pain management.
- The control of pain must be recognised as an important outcome measure in cancer.

References

Department of Health (1998). *A First Class Service: Quality in the new NHS.* London: Department of Health

Finlay IG, Bowdler JM, Tebbit P (2000). *Benchmarking Review of Locally Derived Guidelines on Control of Cancer Pain.* London: National Council for Hospice and Specialist Palliative Care Services

Hearn J & Higginson IJ (1997). Outcome measures in palliative care for advanced cancer patients: a review. *Journal of Public Health Medicine* **19**, 193–199

Higginson IJ, Priest P, McCarthy M (1994). Are bereaved family members a valid proxy for a patient's assessment of dying? *Social Sciences and Medicine* **38**, 553–557

Working Party of the National Council for Hospice and Specialist Palliative Care Services (1995). *Opening Doors: Improving Access to Hospice and Specialist Palliative Care Services by Members of the Black & Ethnic Minority Communities.* London: National Council for Hospice and Specialist Palliative Care Services

Working Party of the National Council for Hospice and Specialist Palliative Care Services (2000). *Positive Partnerships – Palliative Care for Adults with Severe Mental Health problems.* London: National Council for Hospice and Specialist Palliative Care Services

Chapter 10

Developments in general practice and out-of-hours prescribing

Keri Thomas

Introduction

> It was awful – I just panicked! My husband was in agony. It was three o'clock in the morning, we were at home all alone, it was dark and frightening and we didn't know what to do or who to turn to. Things all came together to make his pain seem much worse than it really was.

Pain and fear can be a terrible combination. In our efforts to reduce the burden of cancer pain suffered, we must aim to deliver round-the-clock symptom control in the home as well as in centres of excellence.

The effective delivery of cancer pain services out in the community is determined by the dovetailing of 'generalist palliative care', delivered by general practitioners (GPs) and district nurses (DNs) from the primary healthcare teams (PHCTs), with the available specialist palliative care skills and resources. Those in primary care regard the care of dying patients in the community as an essential and important part of their work. With improvement in cancer therapies and specialist palliative care, more people are living longer, with increasingly complex conditions. There is a movement to increase the numbers of dying people capable of remaining at home, and this presents primary care with a challenge in certain areas, one of them being that of improving the delivery of palliative care out of hours. The aim of this chapter is to outline two areas:

1. Some of the challenges and developments in primary care cancer and palliative care.
2. Out-of-hours palliative care problems, including drug access, and the protocol developed locally in the author's health authority in response.

Cancer and palliative care in general practice

Challenges

It has been estimated that one in three of us will have cancer and one in four will die of it. Most of us are therefore affected by cancer in one way or another at some stage in our lives.

For an average GP with a list size of 2,000 patients, the estimates are that they may have 30–40 patients living with cancer at any one time, about 9 patients newly diagnosed with cancer per year and about 5 or 6 patients dying of cancer per year. Of these, on average two cancer deaths per year will be under the care of the PHCT alone. However, most of the final year of life is spent at home, and the place of care is mainly in the community, no matter where the actual death occurs.

Nationally the death rate at home in England declined with the increase in the number of hospice beds over the last 20 years. Since 1994, with some regional variations, this figure has increased to 26.5%, with the inevitable consequences for primary care (Higginson 1999). Higginson concludes that 'last minute admissions can be inappropriate and distressing' and that 'studying the trends of place of death can help to better understand how to meet the needs of those patients who do wish to be cared for and to die at home'.

With almost half of cancer patients still dying in busy hospital wards and an estimated 22% of hospital bed days taken up by people in the last year of life (Seale & Cartwright 1994), care in the community obviously has a significant impact on secondary services. There can be a tendency towards 'over-institutionalising' and thereby 'over-intervening' in what is essentially a natural process. However, demographic changes mean there are more people without carers, leading to higher and perhaps unrealistic demands that community care would struggle to fulfil. The burden on carers can also be considerable, with chronic fatigue, physical exhaustion, burnout, health deterioration, loss of freedom and financial loss being not uncommon (Stajduhar & Davies 1998). The quality of palliative care in nursing homes and private hospitals is also a major issue.

In his seminal paper on enabling more dying people to remain at home, Thorpe (1993) expressed the following two paradoxes:

1. Most dying people prefer to remain at home but most of them die in institutions.
2. Most of the final year of life is spent at home, but most are admitted to die in hospital.

Thorpe concluded that: 'Not all dying people can be cared for at home and some will choose to die in hospital/hospice. However a large proportion of those admitted could be cared for at home if better support were provided.'

Gomas (1993) felt that returning or keeping a terminally ill patient at home is limited by the instability of the 'patient–family–carer triangle' but that 'palliative care at home embraces what is most noble in medicine: sometimes curing, always relieving, supporting right to the end!'.

A study of palliative care at home in Grampian (Millar *et al.* 1998) looked at the home-based palliative care of 1,086 patients dying of cancer, using a postal questionnaire to GPs and DNs 6 weeks after death. They found the key areas to be symptom control, improved teamwork, further education, communication, use of services and information provision.

Townsend *et al.* (1990) found that, of those dying in hospital, 67% had preferred a home death, and concluded that, with a limited increase in community care, 50% more patients with cancer could be supported to die at home, as they and their carers would have preferred.

There is recognition that expressing a preference for a home death makes it more likely (Karlson & Addington Hall 1998) and that certain groups are more likely to die at home. These include younger patients, those with strong care systems, those of higher socioeconomic status, men, those able to access 24-hour support and those with a shorter trajectory of illness (Higginson 1999). Several studies confirm that symptom control, particularly of pain, may be less than ideal in the community (Addington Hall & McCarthy 1995; Jones *et al.* 1993; Barclay 2000; Hanratty 2000). This was recently reaffirmed in the CancerBACUP Survey (November 2000) of cancer pain, which revealed that:

- 54% of respondents felt they had not been involved in decision-making about pain medication
- 67% of respondents said their doctor had not taken time to discuss with them the different types of pain medication available
- 43% of them had not asked for pain control medication
- 64% of them experienced side effects from their medication
- 10% of them were aware that pain control could be delivered in skin patches.

So, although many are very satisfied with the care that their GP provides, there are still many gaps in the provision of palliative care in the community. Table 10.1 shows some suggested gaps in primary care provision under the three headings of clinical competence, organisational competence and the more nebulous but vitally important area relating to patients' experience of care and our ability to remain human.

Primary care developments

There are many initiatives around the country aiming to improve community palliative care. The recent Beacon Awards in Palliative Care have highlighted many such initiatives, e.g. the Liverpool Integrated Care Pathway for Dying Patients (Ellershaw 1997), which includes care in the last days of life in the community and nursing homes, and Southampton's Resource File, training and education services (R Hillier, personal communication). The Cancer Services Collaborative has pioneered incredible changes in the reorganisation of cancer services in the UK, based on the work of the Institute for Health Care Improvement (Langley *et al.* 1996), and is now extending this to primary care and other specialities – one of the most exciting developments in the NHS today.

Table 10.1 Gaps in community palliative care

1. Clinical competence	1. Assessment of symptoms, e.g. cancer pain
	2. Symptom control and prescribing
	3. Knowing when to refer for specialist help and advice: 'knowing what you don't know'. Continuing education in all areas
2. Organisational competence	4. Communication – information transfer – primary/secondary/specialist palliative care, patient/carer
	5. Access to specialist palliative care/other support, e.g. hospice bed, nightsitters, nursing homes
	6. Co-ordination and continuity, e.g. out-of-hours provision
	7. PHCT workload issues and managed system of care, i.e. ensuring a workable system of care that fits with in with primary care
	8. Social/carer support, e.g. benefits advice, care assistant support, night sitters, etc.
3. Human competence	9. Both patient and carer autonomy and choice.
	10. Listening and communication skills. 'Time to be human' with our patients – getting along and being 'companions on the journey'

Macmillan GP facilitators

There are currently about 60 Macmillan GP facilitators around the UK, who work mainly as experienced GPs with an interest in palliative care, on the boundary between generalist and specialist/secondary care. Overall their aim is to improve the care in the community of cancer and palliative care patients by 'working with GPs and PHCTs and others involved in cancer care in an educational capacity and as agents of change, by mobilising, enhancing and extending existing professional skills' (Thomas & Millar 2000).

The two main goals are therefore to improve education (with practice-based or lecture-style events, newsletters, resource files, etc.) and to act as catalysts of change, attempting to draw people together in responding to the problems raised in discussions with practice teams.

Some facilitators have specialised in the primary care appraisal or accreditation process, setting standards to be attained at all stages of the cancer journey and giving feedback on developmental needs. Many Macmillan GP facilitators have set up initiatives in response to a perceived need of an area, such as out-of-hours palliative care, helplines and formularies. For more details, contact Dr Jane Maher

Chief Medical Officer at Macmillan Cancer Relief (0207 840 4671) or your own Regional Macmillan Office.

Gold standards in community palliative care

In the author's own health authority in West Yorkshire, as Macmillan GP facilitator, inspired by the collaborative approach, she is currently piloting a project looking at six key areas to improve in the care of the dying at home – 'the 6 Cs' – with training, resourcing and an accompanying handbook. The aim is to develop a system or 'toolkit' that is transferable to other practices, is user-friendly and workable in the busy daily life of the PHCT, but that will enable practice teams to aspire to a 'gold standard' of care for their dying patients. These measures should enable improved collaboration, communication and anticipation of needs, with the appropriate harmonising of the generalist skills of the GP and DN with the specialist resources available. The six key tasks are:

- C1   Communication
- C2   Co-ordination
- C3   Control and assessment of symptoms
- C4   Continuity out of hours (see later)
- C5   Continued learning
- C6   Carer support.

Early findings are encouraging as a workable system to bring together many things that teams are already doing, but may not be in a systematised recorded way, which ensures an improved service and a safety net of care. Research suggests that it is often the DN rather than the GP who is the key professional in the community team most in touch with the patients' and carers' needs (Grande *et al.* 1996; Hatcliffe *et al.* 1996; McIlfatrick & Curran 2001), and this project affirms the pivotal role of the DN as co-ordinator of care. (More details, findings and evaluation of this project will be available in summer 2001.)

Palliative care is essentially a primary care issue

Many people feel that, when it comes to dying, 'there's no place like home'. No matter where people actually die, most of the living and dying occurs at home, under the care of the PHCT.

It is my belief that most GPs and DNs work hard to provide good quality care for their dying patients, but would like to be helped to do even better, not by 'specialist take-overs', but by improving the 'speciality of the generalist' in palliative care.

As Pugsley and Pardoe (1986) put it:

> It is never necessary for the team to take over the care of a patient unless that is what the patient and his practitioner wants. It is time that it became recognised that the majority of terminally ill patients are well treated, few are mishandled and only a few cause problems. Perhaps we should remind ourselves that it is better to help a colleague with a difficult case than to tell him he is wrong and that he should make way for the expert.

Marrying the best that primary care has to offer (e.g. relationship, continuity, holistic, context, knowledge of patient and family, etc.) with the expertise of the palliative care specialist (familiarity with conditions, extra knowledge and skills, access to other services, more time, etc.) is a special skill in orchestration.

Out-of-hours palliative care

No discussion about the management of palliative care patients in the community is complete without consideration of out-of-hours care. The perspective here is that from generic primary care, rather than the response of specialist palliative care extending into the community. We have to aim to improve the ordinary care given by out-of-hours providers by dovetailing this with the services provided by specialist centres. The answer to problems out of hours is not necessarily to increase specialist 'hospice at home' or bed availability, useful though this is (Barclay *et al.* 1999), but to empower and upskill the generalist with appropriate help and 24-hour access to advice (Munday & Douglas 1999).

It has been the collective experience of many Macmillan GP facilitators across the country that out-of-hours palliative care in the community can be inadequate, and can lead to inappropriate hospital/hospice admissions and a reduction in the numbers dying at home. No matter how much anticipatory palliative care is provided, there will always be crises, and often these will occur in the 75% of the week outside normal working hours.

It became obvious that, if we are to offer a comprehensive service, we must examine this issue and attempt to address this disparity in accessing care. This was also recognised in *The NHS Cancer Plan* (Milburn 2000) and the *Independent Out of Hours Review* (Department of Health 2000) and the Out of Hours Implementation Group of the Department of Health are currently examining criteria (such as those set out below) for the accreditation of eligibility of out-of-hours providers. The National Association of GP Co-operatives also supports the development of systems to improve care of palliative care patients, as does NHS Direct.

Is out-of-hours care important?

Hanratty and Higginson (1994) stress the importance of continuity of care, believing that emergency visits from strangers are a poor substitute for familiar doctors and nurses. Getting trustworthy, out-of-hours advice is frequently reported as problematic. A recent local survey confirmed that many district nurses believe that out-of-hours availability is a major problem and one of the significant reasons for inappropriate hospital admissions (T Roche, 1999, personal communication). A survey of the views of GPs and DNs revealed that few GPs routinely handed information over to their GP co-operatives, there was much dissatisfaction and that most wanted 24-hour availability of specialist palliative care (Shipman *et al.* 2000).

Winter pressures and Friday discharges exacerbate out-of-hours problems, with an increasing tendency to empty wards before a weekend, sometimes without adequate community back-up. The main reasons for admissions, often inextricably intertwined, are:

- carer breakdown
- symptom control
- communication problems.

For example, the wife who is distressed and anxious about her husband's increasing pain may phone the on-call doctor and regard admission as the only way out. Although studies have shown a preference for home death decreasing as patients approach death (Hinton 1994), the author would argue that on occasions this is not a real choice. If the patient is distressed by difficult symptoms or feels that he or she is a burden to the carer, he or she might accept any option, but this is not a real choice. If symptoms were controlled and the patient and the carers felt well supported and informed, then resorting to admission seems a less likely option. For many, hospices or nursing homes are very appropriate places to die, but few would choose a busy acute hospital ward, after a crisis admission. Although this will inevitably occur in some cases and may often be unavoidable, the fact that almost 50% of our cancer patients die in hospital is still a glaring indictment of our service provision overall. So, the goal of reducing these crisis admissions underpins the requirement to improve out-of-hours palliative care provision.

Changes in GP out-of-hours provision

There have been radical changes in out-of-hours primary care in the last decade, reflecting the unacceptable increase in routine out-of-hours demands. GPs would, on average, have been required to leave their beds on a night visit one night per week in 1994, compared with one night in every 6 weeks in 1967. This form of 24-hour availability has become rare and there has been a shift towards the use of deputising services and GP co-operatives, which has an impact on continuity of care (Salisbury 2000).

Co-operatives have grown across the country, from 30 in 1992 to almost 300 to date, most affiliated to the National Association of GP Co-ops (NAGPC). Healthcall, the country's biggest deputising service, deals with about 18 million people a night.

With the advent of NHS Direct, NHS Direct On Line, NHS Walk-in Centres and the ever-present accident and emergency department, there is less emphasis on general practice as the main point of entry to the NHS. With increasing availability and choice, many feel that quick and convenient access to help may be more important than seeing a doctor they know. The drawbacks, however, include potential confusion, gaps and overlaps, and variability of care. The greatest challenge appears to be in terminally ill people and in those with mental health problems (Salisbury 2000), and many GPs felt that it was their palliative care patients who suffered most with the advent of these changes. As one cancer patient put it:

> . . . a Bank Holiday weekend can feel like a long dark tunnel without the lifeline of
> help at the end of the phone.

Patients or carers using a co-operative/deputising service may see many different doctors and nurses, with the painful repetition of their story (e.g. 11 different co-operative clinicians over one weekend). Crisis visits from strangers unfamiliar with their details, with little knowledge of how to deal with different palliative care situations or how to access help, and with difficulties accessing appropriate drugs can lead to a lack of trust and confidence in their primary care cover. Consequently, more reliance may be placed on the specialists who pick up the pieces, thereby altering the focus of care away from home.

Therefore improvements in co-ordination, quality assurance, accessibility of information, support and drugs have never been more vital in the care of those with life-threatening illness at home.

Hospices provide an outstanding service, but are often over-stretched and under-staffed, with many consultants doing permanent on-call for the community patients, patching up the gaps in primary care. However, with better generic resourcing and co-ordination of primary care out of hours for those most in need, hospice resources could be better directed.

Possible solutions

The problems in out-of-hours care seem to fall into a framework of four main areas (Thomas 2000):

- communication problems
- reduced access to support services
- reduced access to medical advice
- reduced access to drugs and equipment.

As Macmillan GP facilitator in her own area, the author sought the views of all involved in out-of-hours palliative care, including primary care groups, district nursing services, local medical committees, pharmaceutical advisers, the newly developed doctors' co-operative and the longstanding deputising service Healthcall. Her group devised a 4-point plan (Table 10.2) which involved only three new initiatives (the Handover Form, Bearder Bags and Crisis Pack), but was mainly a drawing together and co-ordinating of pre-existing services, with dissemination of information.

Table 10.2 Four-point action plan (Calderdale & Kirklees' Out Of Hours Protocol)

1. Communication	(a) use handover form – GP/DN – send to on-call service and keep in DN notes?
	(b) inform others, e.g. hospice?
	(c) does the carer know what to do in a crisis?
2. Carer support	(a) co-ordinate pre-emptive care, e.g. nightsitters, 24-hour DN
	(b) give written information to carers
	(c) emergency support, e.g. rapid response team
3. Medical support	(a) anticipated management in handover form
	(b) crisis pack, guidelines, etc. and ongoing teaching
	(c) 24-hour specialist advice available from hospice
4. Drugs/equipment	(a) leave anticipated drugs in home
	(b) Bearder palliative care bags in co-op cars
	(c) on-call stocked pharmacists

The Handover Form was piloted and then reviewed by a team of GPs and specialists involving NHS Direct, who were triaging all local calls to the co-operative. It is completed by the GP/DN, faxed to the co-op or Healthcall to inform the visiting on-call doctor, and kept in the DN's notes in the patient's home. With the advent of electronic transfer of information (electronic health records, etc.) this will soon become even easier. The Handover Form has two vitally important functions: first, to transfer information about the patient's diagnosis, management plan, treatment and particular needs, e.g. wishes to remain at home, GP would like to be called at home, etc. Second, to build in proactive planning, e.g. if the GP/DN completing the form considers that the patient may need a certain drug, such as midazolam or hyoscine, then the form acts as a trigger to leave the drugs in the patient's home, with appropriate authorisation.

Support services to prevent carer breakdown improved with the development of 24-hour district nursing across the whole patch, and a generic rapid response team, to support carers with care assistants if a hospital admission was otherwise inevitable.

Medical support was improved by the transmission of the GP's plan of care via the Handover Form, a crisis pack of 'at the bedside' guidelines backed up by specific training sessions for doctors doing a call. Also, the availability of advice from palliative care doctors at the two hospices was co-ordinated and better advertised, so the visiting on-call doctor felt more comfortable phoning for advice out of hours.

Problems with drug access out of hours

Three measures seek to address this problem:

- The first stage is to encourage GPs to leave the anticipated drugs in the home, prompted by the Handover Form (routine drugs allowing for dose increases or use of commonly used 'end-stage' drugs for the on-call doctor or DN to use).
- The second measure was to stock on-call pharmacists with an agreed list of palliative care drugs (costing under £100) and a central number to co-ordinate the on-call rota, allowing health professionals access to these pharmacists (some other areas have formed their own on-call rota via the local pharmaceutical committee).
- The third addition is the use of a palliative care bag, stocked with palliative care drugs. A local charitable trust, founded by John Bearder, donated funds to help prevent further problems with drug access in the terminal stages. These contain all the predicted drugs that might be required for palliative care patients, a syringe driver and other equipment, along with crisis packs containing guidelines and contact phone numbers. They are kept in the co-op cars or at Healthcall base.

One of the recommendations of *The Independent Out-of-Hours Review* (2000) is that patients should be able to receive the medication they need at the same time and in the same place as the out-of-hours consultation, i.e. the visiting doctor should be able to have all the drugs required at the time of the consultation.

If regulations change accordingly this will be a considerable help to many, the author's group included, especially regarding controlled drugs and access to the very necessary opioid analgesics, such as diamorphine, that our terminal patients require. However, in the light of the post-Shipman debate, strict regulations are likely to follow, although a sensible balance must be reached between prevention of abuse and ease of access to those in need.

There are some particular problems with controlled drugs, i.e.

- storage of controlled drugs and Home Office regulations
- prescribing and logging of stock
- transport (UKCC regulations do allow nurses to transport controlled drugs but only in exceptional circumstances)
- leaving controlled drugs in the home – these ought to be in locked containers to prevent abuse
- accessing controlled drugs from hospices – hospices are not considered as authorised dispensers to the community so, although this source has been used, it is not to be recommended.

It is hoped that, if changes in the regulations are brought into effect, access to diamorphine will be made easier for terminal patients, and the difficulties many have faced will be overcome.

As one carer put it:

> Your main concern is the PAIN that is being suffered. Pain is no respector of class or creed .... Pain is pain and it doesn't go away. Filling in forms doesn't do that, but organising systems and filling in forms may help to alleviate and prevent that suffering.

Along with the author's local palliative care consultants, several training sessions have been run for out-of-hours doctors, going through the usage of the drugs in the Bearder bags, the guidelines, case histories and the availability of 24-hour specialist advice via the hospices. Many GPs were unhappy about the use of some 'unusual' drugs, e.g. midazolam, methotrimeprazine. Also, several did not feel confident about setting up a syringe driver at 3am, under stressful circumstances. It was agreed that, rather than struggling with the unfamiliar complexities of syringe drivers, the on-call doctor should alleviate the symptom with a subcutaneous stat dose of, for example, diamorphine, which would allow 4 hours in which the DN could set up the syringe driver. Other areas, perhaps more rural, have made different decisions. The relief from the on-call doctors was almost palpable and confidence in their ability to cope rose enormously! (The Calderdale & Kirklees Health Authority out-of-hours palliative care protocol is currently being independently evaluated in both qualitative and quantitative research and findings and conclusions will be available from August 2001.)

Macmillan out-of-hours report

This Report is a distillation of the views, experiences and solutions from Macmillan GP facilitators and many others involved in out-of-hours palliative care around the country. With extensive consultation, an open forum, redrafting and much further consultation, a substantial report was drawn up, with specific recommendations relating to out-of-hours palliative care in the community. The appendix also contains several examples of good practice and templates for others to use. The Report has been available from Macmillan Cancer Relief since March 2001.

Conclusions

In this chapter some of the challenges and developments in primary care relevant to the treatment of cancer pain in palliative care have been briefly described.

Some of the problems of out-of-hours palliative care and access to drugs have been outlined and the approach taken in response in the author's health authority described. The Macmillan Report on Out of Hours Palliative Care in the community, which outlines several other approaches, has also been alluded to.

We now live in an era of the 'primary care-led NHS'. The author is confident that small changes can make a great impact, that organising and improving systems will make a real difference, and that primary care can meet the challenges that face us in the future with the care of our dying patients at home, so that we too can say that 'palliative care at home embraces what is most noble in medicine: sometimes curing, always relieving, supporting right to the end' (Gomas 1993).

References

Addington-Hall J & McCarthy M (1995). Dying from cancer: results of a national population-based investigation. *Palliative Medicine* **9**, 295–305

Barclay S (2000). The management of cancer pain in primary care. *The Effective Management of Cancer Pain*. London: Aesculapius Medical Press, pp 117–129

Barclay SI, Todd C, McCabe J, Hunt T (1999). Primary Care groups commissioning of services: the differing priorities of general practitioners and district nurses for palliative care services. *British Journal of General Practice* **49**, 181–186

Department of Health (2000). *Independent Out of Hours Review*. London: DoH

Ellershaw J (1997). Developing an integrated care pathway for the dying patient. *European Journal of Palliative Care* **4**, 203–207

Gomas J-M (1993). Palliative care at home: a reality or 'mission impossible'? *Palliative Medicine* **7**(suppl 11), 45–59

Grande GE, Todd CJ, Barclay SIG, Doyle JH (1996). What terminally patients value in the support provided by GPs district and Macmillan nurses. *International Journal of Palliative Medicine* **2**, 138–143

Hanratty B (2000). Palliative Care provided by GPs: the carer's viewpoint. *British Journal of General Practice* **50**, 653–654

Hanratty J & Higginson I (1994). *Palliative Care in Terminal Illness*. Oxford: Radcliffe Medical Press

Hatcliffe S, Smith P, Daw R (1996). District nurses' perceptions of palliative care at home. *Nursing Times* **92**, 36–37

Higginson I (1999). Evidence based palliative care. *British Medical Journal* **319**, 462–463

Higginson IJ, Astin P, Dolan S (1998). Where do cancer patients die? Ten year trends in the place of death of cancer patients in England. *Palliative Medicine* **12**, 353

Hinton J (1994). Can home care maintain an acceptable quality of life for patients with terminal cancer and their relatives? *Palliative Medicine* **8**, 183–196

Jones R, Hansford J, Fiske J (1993). Death from cancer at home: the carer's perspective. *British Medical Journal* **306**, 249–251

Karlson, Addington Hall J (1998). How do cancer patients who die at home differ from those who die elsewhere? *Palliative Medicine* **12**, 279–284

Langley G, Nolan K, Nolan T *et al.* (1996*). The Improvement Guide. A practical approach to enhancing organisational performance*. San Francisco: Jossey Bass Publishers

McIlfatrick S & Curran C (2001). The perceived role of the DN in palliative care. *Journal of Community Nursing* **15**, in press

Millar DG, Carroll D, Grimshaw J, Watt B (1998). Palliative care at home: an audit of cancer deaths in Grampian region. *British Journal of General Practice* **48**, 1299–1302

Milburn A (2000). *The NHS Cancer Plan*. London: Department of Health

Munday D, Douglas A, Carroll D (1999). GP out of hours co-operatives and the delivery of palliative care. *British Journal of General Practice* **49**, 489

Pugsley R & Pardoe J (1986). The specialist contribution to the care of the terminally ill patient: support or substitution? *Journal of Royal College of General Practitioners* 347–348

Salisbury C (2000). Out of hours care: ensuring accessible high quality care for all groups of patients. *British Journal of General Practice* **50**, 443–444

Seale C & Cartwright A (1994). *The Year before Death*. Aldershot: Avebury

Shipman C, Addington-Hall J, Barclay S *et al.* (2000). Providing palliative care in primary care: how satisfied are GPs and district nurses with current out of hours arrangements? *British Journal of General Practice* **50**, 477–478

Stajduhar KI & Davies B (1998). Death at home challenges for families and directions for the future. *Journal of Palliative Care* **14**, 8–14

Thomas K (2000). Out of hours palliative care – bridging the gap. *European Journal of Palliative Care* **7**, 22–25

Thomas K & Millar D (2000). Catalysts for change. *Palliative Care Today*

Thorpe G (1993). Enabling more dying people to remain at home. *British Medical Journal* **307**, 915–918

Townsend J, Frank AO, Fermont D *et al.* (1990). Terminal cancer care and patients' preference for place of death. *British Medical Journal* **301**, 415–417

Increasing the effectiveness of intervention through multidisciplinary models of care: the nature of nurse-led intervention

Anne Lanceley

Introduction

The WHO, international and national professional organisations and governments have, for some time, advanced the critical importance of pain management as an essential part of cancer care. Yet for large numbers of people with cancer their pain 'remains inadequately treated' (Foley 1999). Studies using a variety of methods and that have included patients with advanced or far advanced disease demonstrate a prevalence of pain in between 58% and 84% of patients (Hearn & Higginson 1999). Late-stage cancer is associated with more pain than earlier stages, but Portenoy and Lesage (1999) reported that chronic pain is experienced by about 30–40% of cancer patients undergoing treatment for solid tumours. Prospective studies have indicated that up to 90% of patients could attain adequate relief with simple drug therapies, but this success rate is not borne out in practice (Teoh & Stjernsward 1992; Portenoy *et al.* 1994).

Barriers to the treatment of cancer pain include a variety of complex educational, attitudinal and institutional obstacles, e.g. there appears to be a deficiency in the pain assessment and management training of both doctors and nurses, a tendency in some clinical settings to give lower priority to symptom control than to disease management, and a belief that symptoms are best managed by establishing their underlying cause and by utilising modern pharmacological and biomedical innovations for their relief (Breitbart *et al.* 1998).

Explanations for the continued inadequate management of pain in cancer are complex, and this is perhaps reflected in a recent survey of UK patients with cancer undertaken by CancerBACUP, the national cancer information charity. Despite the growing recognition of the need for healthcare professional/patient partnerships in healthcare decision-making (Department of Health 1998), 54% of the 157 survey participants said that they had not been sufficiently involved in decision-making about their treatment for pain (Mayor 2000). Other studies reveal that, despite patients reporting frequent communication regarding pain and pain control with doctors, nurses and pharmacists, this had not dispelled their stoicism and fatalism in the face of their pain which represented a significant barrier to pain control (Riddell & Fitch 1997; Thomason *et al.* 1998). In the study by Thomason *et al.* (1998), 88% of the 239 participants ranked their pain as 5 or greater on a visual analogue scale, and 81% reported impaired function as a result of pain.

In the turbulent world of health care, it is not sufficient to increase individual knowledge and learning about cancer pain management. The assimilation of individual knowledge into new organisational and team work structures, routines and norms is essential to develop approaches to pain management in which the individual and their own understanding is at the centre of the therapeutic intervention.

Although the central place of the patient in their care is recognised at government policy level (Department of Health 2000a), debated in the professional literature (Corner & Dunlop 1997) and accepted as a fundamental tenant of cancer and palliative care pain management practice (Saunders 1967; World Health Organization 1990), the extent and nature of the change needed truly to realise this in practice have been underestimated (Bell *et al.* 1996) It is, for example, accepted that the effective treatment of cancer pain depends on a comprehensive assessment, which, according to Portenoy and Lesage (1999), characterises the pain in terms of: 'phenomenology and pathogenesis, assesses the relation between the pain and the disease, and clarifies the impact of the pain and co-morbid conditions on the patients quality of life'. It is an approach that demands that the healthcare professional actively and consistently negotiates with cancer pain sufferers to create situations which can interpret, alleviate and 'contain' the pain (Lanceley 1995), as well as assess the need for powerful drugs, and it begs the question of who, in the healthcare team, is best placed to do this.

This chapter analyses evidence for the nature and effectiveness of nurse-led interventions in health care and extrapolates the limited findings to cancer pain management, from diagnosis to treatment, rehabilitation and through to palliative care. The potential impact of nurse-led interventions on the roles and responsibilities of other multidisciplinary team members is considered. The chapter is informed by significant policy directives in cancer services, together with an analysis of gaps in knowledge that may impede the effective management of cancer pain as envisioned in the current policy context.

Policy context

A reassessment and revaluation of professional roles and core values is identified in the *NHS Cancer Plan* (Department of Health 2000a) as a key trend across health professions, involving redistribution of the tasks undertaken by members of various caring professions, and a move towards blurring of professional boundaries. The professional bodies have been keen to describe the particular skills that different health professionals bring to bear on solving health problems, e.g. the General Medical Council's revised edition of *Good Medical Practice* (General Medical Council 1998) recognises the importance of clinical teams and acknowledges a change in the relationship between doctors and other healthcare staff. The Royal

Colleges of Radiologists and Radiographers (1998) have used the principles established in the GMC's document to prepare their own statement, *Inter-professional Roles and Responsibilities in a Clinical Oncology Service*. A further document encouraging the constructive development of skills mix in cancer care is the joint report of the Royal College of Radiologists, the Royal College of Nursing and the College of Radiographers (Board of the Faculty of Clinical Oncology 1999).

The role of nurses in cancer care was specifically highlighted in *A Policy Framework for Commissioning Cancer Services* (Calman & Hine 1995), which advocates models of collaborative, interdisciplinary working and recognises the crucial role nurses play in the delivery of a comprehensive cancer service. The current Department of Health debate on extending nurse prescribing is an outworking of this and is highly relevant to this discussion about nurse-led interventions for cancer pain management. Under the most radical option being proposed, all general sales lists and pharmacy medicines prescribable on the NHS list, including controlled drugs, would be added to the *Nurse Prescribers' Formulary*. Specialist cancer and palliative care nurses who successfully complete prescribing education courses would be able to prescribe legally and this right would be determined by patient need and discussion with employers (Department of Health 2001).

The Nursing Contribution to Cancer Care (Department of Health 2000b) explores the possibilities and benefits to patients of nurses collaborating with members of the interprofessional team to pioneer new ways of working. In addition to recognising the frontline position of nurses dealing with anxieties and uncertainties of patients in pain and their families, this strategic document identifies the need to:

- build and use the evidence base to support and inform cancer nursing interventions
- evaluate the effectiveness of new nursing roles.

Although acknowledging that cancer nurses have a strong orientation to quality improvement, the document also points out that education for specialist nurse roles in cancer care is patchy or non-existent. In addition, it states that 'More evidence is needed about the relationship between care practices and interventions and patient outcomes and investment is needed in continuing professional development to promote the skills necessary to foster evidence-based cancer nursing'. Increasingly, therefore, the distinctive role of nursing is being explored and there is some evidence in cancer and other areas of practice, of the effectiveness of nurse interventions, of team systems led by nurses, or elements of service provision being 'nurse-led'. (There are no exact criteria for identifying services as nurse-led (Garbett 1996). Common features are nurse autonomy in admitting and discharging patients, together with the authority to make decisions within the remit of the service, e.g. in the case of altering a drug dose.)

The evidence base for the effectiveness of nurse-led interventions

Four trials published recently in the *British Medical Journal* of practice nurses' interventions for self-limiting minor illnesses are cases in point, and give us a good idea of what the future of primary care might look like. Although the clinical focus on minor illnesses, the small sample sizes and the short follow-up of 2 weeks in three of the studies is open to criticism, the studies nevertheless raise important questions (Kinnersley *et al.* 2000; Lattimer *et al.* 2000; Shum *et al.* 2000; Venning *et al.* 2000). If, as the studies demonstrated, on average nurses have longer consultations, arrange more investigations and follow-up, provide more information and give more satisfaction than general practitioners, what roles should primary care nurses occupy and what contribution could they make to cancer patients' pain management? Does their future lie in case management of patients along care pathways and in organising and coordinating team care?

In 1991, McMahon and Pearson published their book *Nursing as Therapy*, which is founded on the belief that a certain form of nursing, involving deliberate nurse decision-making, has a powerful effect on the patient and promotes adaptation, healing and health. Areas in which nursing was considered to have therapeutic potential were the nurse–patient relationship, the interpersonal care environment, providing comfort, conventional and unconventional nursing interventions, and patient teaching.

Empirical evidence for McMahon and Pearson's assertions about the therapeutic potential of nursing is a multi-centre randomised controlled trial to evaluate the effectiveness of nursing intervention for breathlessness in patients with lung cancer (Bredin *et al.* 1999). Patients with lung cancer either attended a nursing clinic offering intervention for their breathlessness or received 'best supportive care'. The intervention consisted of: a range of strategies combining assessment of breathlessness and factors that ameliorate or exacerbate it; advice and support plus goal setting for sufferers and their families on ways of managing breathlessness, including breathing re-training techniques, activity pacing, relaxation techniques and psychosocial support; and the early recognition of problems warranting biomedical intervention. An important facet of the intervention was the exploration of the meaning of the breathlessness, the disease and feelings about the future by specialist cancer nurses together with the patients. Best supportive care involved receiving standard management and treatment available for breathlessness, combined with breathing assessments. Patients who attended the nursing clinics and received the breathlessness intervention experienced improvement in breathlessness, performance status, and physical and emotional states relative to control patients, thus confirming findings from an earlier study (Corner *et al.* 1996). Despite being open to some criticisms (the analysis assumes that patients who withdrew had a poor outcome; patients whose baseline measurements were at the extremes of the rating scale could show change in only one direction and, although differences between the two groups of patients were significant, the magnitude of the effect of the intervention was more difficult to assess), the study makes a significant contribution to evaluating the nursing contribution to symptom management by bringing out the focused, patient-need-driven, purposefully emotional work of nurses in relationship with patients.

Another example of nurses responding to a symptom of cancer illness as a need or problem unique to an individual is the work of Krishnasamy (2000) to develop new multi-professional approaches to the management of fatigue in advanced cancer. This quasi-experimental study set out to assess the feasibility of an intervention designed to minimise the distress experienced by patients and their relatives by:

- maximising functional capacity through harnessing and promoting energy resources
- prioritising daily routines
- providing a supportive environment within which to explore and discuss fears and anxieties.

This approach is delivered in a nurse-led clinic setting, during group sessions led by the multi-professional team. Outcome measures include a series of visual analogue scales measuring distress, presence of pain, degree of loss of concentration, night sleeping pattern and perception of loss of energy at its worst and best. In addition the WHO functional capacity measure, a fatigue subscale, a measure of the effects of serious illness, and a quality of life instrument have been used to evaluate the intervention. The co-ordinated programme of care, including nurse, occupational therapy and physiotherapy support, took place over a 5-week period in a day-care hospice setting. Patients suffering from fatigue benefited from this approach and strategies employed in the study warrant further multi-centre research.

Another example of a nurse-led intervention is the work of Preston (1995) on the management of malignant ascites. The starting point for this work is that ascites is a form of lymphoedema, so a self-management strategy is proposed based on principles of lymphoedema management. Optimal ways of delaying reaccumulation of ascites are currently being tested in women with ovarian cancer. The women are taught to increase the pressure in their abdomen throughout the day through breathing exercise regimens, as well as wearing an abdominal binder, in order to optimise their remaining lymphatic channels. Nurse-led services for the management of lymphoedema have been in existence for a decade or more, and this work is an extension of this.

In addition to studies exploring the role of nursing in innovations in clinical practice, there is a growing body of evidence for nursing's contribution to reconfigured services, e.g. traditional follow-up of cancer patients after treatment is an expensive and time-consuming focus of clinical activity, and it is increasingly recognised that this may not benefit the patient in terms of survival, quality of life or specifically facilitating patients to talk about their pain or other symptoms (Brada 1995). A study by Rogers and Todd (2000) demonstrates this. The study revealed, through qualitative analysis of communication between cancer patients and oncologists during consultations in outpatient clinics, that doctors tightly control the agenda to focus narrowly on pain that is amenable to radiotherapy, chemotherapy, surgery or hormone manipulation. Although pain is a problem reported in more than half of the outpatient oncology consultations, and talk about pain occupies a substantial proportion of each consultation (22%), oncologists routinely sought information to make treatment decisions and gave little attention to patients' reports of pain and its impact on their lives – a finding that is consistent with the recent CancerBACUP patient survey mentioned earlier and a postal survey designed to elicit the relatives' perspective on pain relief (Miettinen *et al.* 1998).

There is growing evidence for the effectiveness of nurse-led follow-up clinics for cancer patients (James *et al.* 1994; McArdle *et al.* 1996; Earnshaw & Stephensen 1997; Stiggelbout *et al.* 1997; Faithfull 1999; Campbell *et al.* 2000). The study by Rogers and Todd (2000) legitimates re-thinking follow-up services and pioneering different ways of working with patients experiencing pain.

Earnshaw and Stephensen (1997) report on the first 2 years of a follow-up breast clinic led by a nurse practitioner. The nurse-led clinic proved popular with patients. Appointments were longer than in the general clinic and women perceived that the nurse had time to discuss their concerns about their prosthesis, lymphoedema, and tamoxifen therapy. Self-management strategies were taught and women learned breast self-examination and received general advice and information about ongoing clinical trials. The nurse offered patients the opportunity of a joint interview with their partner or another person close to them, helped patients to express feelings and listened sympathetically to sexual difficulties and feelings of inadequacy. A concern that some breast cancer recurrences will not be detected by the nurse practitioner was not borne out in practice. These findings are consistent with results from a questionnaire survey eliciting patient satisfaction with clinical nurse specialists in a breast care clinic by Garvican *et al.* (1998).

The examples of successful nurse-led interventions described above share principles in common, notably:

- Rigorous assessment based on the patient's narrative of their experience of the symptom, alongside other assessment data
- Care starts from the perspective of the patient
- Interventions are designed to foster personhood and control, and to acknowledge suffering and distress, and the central importance of individual meaning to the experience of cancer illness.

As Corner and Dunlop (1997) point out, how patients view symptoms is crucial to developing effective symptom management. In the studies reviewed, nurses were clearly effective in eliciting patients' views and working with them to deal with their symptoms over time. A significant aspect of the nurses work with the patients in the studies described is how the nurse uses her capacity to perceive and interpret the subjective experience of the patient. What is needed now is the development of nurse-led care programmes that combine pharmacological and non-pharmacological approaches – work that is currently in its infancy (Carroll & Seers 1998; Seers & Carroll 1998). There is an additional type of evidence concerning individual expression of pain that may be significant in informing the development of nurse-led initiatives in cancer pain management.

It is the essential inexpressibility and indeterminate nature of pain which presents such a challenge to healthcare professionals concerned to help patients with their pain according to Scarry (1985) and Kleinman et al. (1992). What is of interest to these researchers is how people attribute meaning to their pain. Kleinman, a medical anthropologist, noted how patients will attempt to order the experience of their pain, what it means to them and those close to them, through personal narratives of their illness. These stories are not fixed, but are constantly being told and retold. There is a sense in which the narratives not only reflect experience but create it. This is achieved by the story lines and key metaphors and rhetorical devices chosen by the patient in their oft times desperate attempts to make sense of their pain and describe it to others.

In a series of recent articles, Greenhalgh and Hurwitz (1999) have recommended working with patient narratives in the management of chronic illness, and Greenhalgh cites her work with patients with diabetes. There is potential for narrative-based cancer pain management strategies to supplement and enrich our biomedical knowledge with the personal and cultural meanings patients carve out of pain, e.g. existing multidimensional pain assessment tools may be supplemented by patient profiles and diaries.

Jackson (1994) makes an important observation in her study of people with chronic pain and one that may also be relevant to developing care programmes: that patients in pain attempt to manipulate subject/object distinctions for their own therapeutic good. In her study patients sought relief from their chronic pain, both by intensive subjectification of the pain – 'I believe the snake (i.e. the pain) is me' or 'My God I was afraid of it but the pain is me' – or by increased objectification when the pain is referred to as an 'it' and something entirely separate from their body and self. The urgent need to try to explain and find meaning in the pain experience may be at the root of the patients' attempts to first invoke then blur the subject–object distinctions inherent in our dualistic separation of mind from body.

Sontag (1991) first gave prominence to the idea that metaphor plays a significant role in the construction of cancer illness. The metaphorical potency of cancer illness is recognised by a number of writers (Di Giacomo 1987; Stacey 1997) and there is significant empirical evidence within the broad field of health and illness research that patients routinely use metaphor to express their feelings (Jenny & Logan 1996; Radley 1993). More recent work (Lanceley 1999) demonstrates that cancer patients consistently use metaphor to give expression to the demands made upon them by their illness. The pursuit of metaphorical expression of feeling in this study of nurse–patient conversations revealed important ways in which patients use metaphors not only as vehicles for the expression of hidden feelings, but as a protection against them. Metaphors allowed the patients to approach the truth of their illness obliquely, which was perhaps less threatening to them, and to the nurse. This finding raises important questions for the interprofessional team in developing new approaches to the management of cancer pain. If the patient conceives cancer pain and treatment metaphorically, it may be that the symptom is best coped with and responded to by healthcare professionals in this way. Questions arise as to how nurses might work with patients in interpreting their metaphors and developing understanding. It is perhaps unlikely that we will achieve patient-centred care if we deny patients their individual metaphoric interpretation of their illness. However, empirical studies will be needed to evaluate the potential benefits of interpretative responses to cancer patients' metaphors.

It seems from the evidence presented that effective nurse-led approaches in cancer pain management are likely to be those that are focused and involve collaboration with the patient to address the emotional and sociocultural aspects of their pain purposefully. Longitudinal studies that examine these processes in cancer and palliative care are urgently needed, but what are the first steps in establishing these principles for practice?

The way forward?

There is enthusiasm among cancer care professionals for consideration of the value of management approaches from other clinical settings in oncology practice (Morris 1996; Selwood 2000). The integrated pathway approach is one that deserves clinical champions, if only for the fact that patients need to be widely consulted in order that their experiences can be used as legitimate sources of evidence on which to base practice.

Lessons from integrated pathway methodology may be useful in deciding and formalising new roles and responsibilities of team members in the management of cancer pain. Pathways are identified by Currie and Harvey (2000) as 'a way of improving quality through embedding evidence into practice', using this evidence to develop pathways which detail the essential steps in the care of patients with a specific clinical problem or symptom, and analysing data on variation to improve practice.

Since pathway plans define and detail medical, nursing and therapy interventions, they have the potential to help in communication with patients by giving them access to a clearly written summary of their expected care plan and progress over time (Sulch & Kalra 2000). This view is supported by the study by Currie and Harvey (2000), which explored the experiences and views of a range of healthcare professionals using care pathways in their everyday practice. Currie and Harvey also found that integrated pathway records can improve understanding of the roles of different disciplines and promote teamwork in patient care, a finding supported by Campbell *et al.* (1998).

The majority of care pathways have been developed for acute illness episodes and are *condition* or *procedure* specific, leading to some scepticism about their use in managing patient problems such as pain that are characterised by unpredictability and complexity. It can be argued that the inherent linear, more rational–deductive assumptions in integrated care pathways – that care can be standardised – do not hold true for cancer pain management and that, as a tool for multiprofessional working, pathways would be difficult to generate and have little to offer the range of practitioners involved in managing cancer pain. After all, the process of cancer pain management cannot begin or end with a discrete therapeutic event and it is rarely clearly defined or possible to plot expected progress in pain control over time. In addition interdisciplinary practice is well established in oncology and palliative care units, and at first it may seem that integrated care pathways may have little further to contribute.

Although there is a lack of robust evidence of the effectiveness of integrated care pathways in cancer care, some evidence exists in support of specific elements which make up the integrated pathway approach and these have the potential to improve the care of cancer patients in pain. For example, the development of a pathway based on current or best practice stimulates critical questioning and appraisal of practice in order to make decisions and reach a consensus about the content of the pathway (Middleton & Roberts 2000). Practitioners involved in 'working up' a pathway also have to consider the types of evidence they will use to inform it. Research-based evidence, experiential evidence – often the accumulation of years of clinical expertise – and evidence derived directly from patients' experience can all be used as a basis to inform the development of a pathway (Rossiter & Thompson 1995). Another valuable element of the approach is that, in cases where developing a pathway highlights gaps in the evidence base, the systematic auditing and careful recording of variance from the pathway helps generate evidence to support a particular intervention (Kitchiner *et al.* 1996).

Conclusions

This chapter has considered evidence for how the multidisciplinary team may further understand and work with the needs of patients and their families to manage their cancer pain. Processes that foster personhood and acknowledge chronicity, distress and meaning as fundamental to the experience of having cancer and being in pain are seen as the key to improving the management of cancer pain. Where nurse-led interventions may be most useful is in the process of pain management. The nurses' interactions with patients in this case may be characterised by a different language, beyond the objective and factual. Comparative studies will be needed to evaluate different kinds of approaches that go hand in hand with excellent pharmacological management.

If cancer patients are to be effectively helped with their pain and services refocused to meet their needs and expectations, it is essential to analyse the different functions of multidisciplinary team members. Integrated care pathway approaches offer a way of doing this, for evidence-based guidelines may be woven into a new pattern of interactions and values where the roles of team members are clearly delineated and the nature and range of interventions associated with each role agreed by the team and formalised. The potential is huge for the rigorous evaluation of such care programmes and the communication of good and innovative models of practice.

References

Bell S, Brada M, Coombes C *et al.* (1996). Patient-*centred services? What patients say.* Oxford: National Cancer Alliance

Board of the Faculty of Clinical Oncology (1999). *Skills Mix in Clinical Oncology.* London: Royal College of Radiologists

Brada M (1995). Is there a need to follow-up cancer patients? *European Journal of Cancer and Clinical Oncology* **31A**, 655–657

Bredin M, Corner J, Krishnasamy M *et al.* (1999). Multicentre randomised controlled trial of nursing intervention for breathlessness in patients with lung cancer. *British Medical Journal* **318**, 901–904

Breitbart W, Rosenfeld B, Passik SD (1998). The network project: A multidisciplinary cancer education and training program in pain management, rehabilitation, and psychosocial issues. *Journal of Pain and Symptom Management* **15**, 18–26

Calman K & Hine D (1995). *A Policy Framework for Commissioning Cancer Services.* Department of Health, Wales

Campbell H, Hotchkiss R, Bradshaw N *et al.* (1998). Integrated care pathways. *British Medical Journal* **316**, 133–137

Campbell J, German L, Lane C (2000). Radiotherapy outpatient review: A nurse-led clinic. *Clinical Oncology* **12**, 104–107

Carroll D & Seers K (1998). Relaxation for the relief of chronic pain: a systematic review. *Journal of Advanced Nursing* **27**, 476–487

Corner J & Dunlop R (1997). New approaches to care. In Clark D, Hockley J, Ahmedzai S (eds) *New Themes in Palliative Care.* Buckingham: Open University Press, pp 288–302

Corner J, Plant H, Alhern R *et al.* (1996). Non-pharmacological intervention for breathlessness in lung cancer. *Palliative Medicine* **10**, 299–305

Currie VL & Harvey G (2000). The use of care pathways as tools to support the implementation of evidence based practice. *Journal of Interprofessional Care* **14**, 311–323

Department of Health (1998). *Putting Patients First.* London: Department of Health

Department of Health (2000a). *The NHS Cancer Plan.* London: Department of Health

Department of Health (2000b). *The Nursing Contribution to Cancer Care: A strategic programme of action in support of the national cancer programme.* London: Department of Health

Department of Health (2001). *Extended Prescribing of Prescription Only Medicines by Independent Nurse Prescribers.* Consultation Document. London: Department of Health

Di Giacomo SM. (1987). Biomedicine as a cultural system; An anthropologist in the kingdom of the sick. In Baer H (ed.) *Encounters in Biomedicine: Case studies in medical anthropology* New York: Gordon & Breach, pp 315–346

Earnshaw JJ & Stephensen Y (1997) First year of a follow -up breast clinic led by a nurse practitioner. *Journal of the Royal Society of Medicine* **90**, 258–259

Faithfull S (1999) Randomized trial, a method of comparisons: a study of supportive care in radiotherapy nursing. *European Journal of Oncology Nursing* **3** (3) 176–184

Foley KM (1999). Advances in cancer pain. *Archives of Neurology* **56**, 1–9

Garbett R (1996). The growth of nurse-led care. *Nursing Times* **92**, 29

Garvican LE, Grimsey E, Littlejohns P *et al.* (1998). Satisfaction with clinical nurse specialists in a breast care clinic. *British Medical Journal* **316**, 976–977

General Medical Council (1998). *Good Medical Practice.* London: General Medical Council

Greenhalgh T & Hurwitz B (1999). Narrative based medicine: Why study narrative? *British Medical Journal* **318**, 48–50

Hearn J & Higginson IJ (1999). *Epidemiology of Pain: Pain associated with cancer.* Task Force on Epidemiology. Seattle: International Association for the Study of Pain

Jackson J (1994). Chronic pain and the tension between the body as subject and object. In Csordas TB (ed.) *Embodiment and Experience: The existential ground of culture and self.* Cambridge: Cambridge University Press, pp 201–228

James ND, Guerreo D, Brada M (1994). Who should follow up cancer patients? Nurse specialist based outpatient care and the introduction of a phone clinic system. *Clinical Oncology* **6**, 283–287

Jenny J & Logan J (1996). Caring and comfort metaphors used by patients in critical care. *Image: Journal of Nursing Scholarship* **28**, 349–352

Kinnersley P, Anderson E, Parry K *et al.* (2000). Randomised controlled trial of nurse practitioner versus general practitioner care for patients requesting 'same day' consultations in primary care. *British Medical Journal* **320**, 1043–1048

Kitchiner D, Davidson C, Bundred P (1996). Integrated care pathways: effective tools for continuous evaluation of clinical practice. *Journal of Evaluation in Clinical Practice* **2**, 65–69

Kleinman A *et al.* (1992). Pain as human experience: an introduction. In DelVecchio Good M-J, Good B, Kleinman A (eds) *Pain as Human Experience.* Berkeley: University of California Press, pp 1–27

Krishnasamy M (2000). Fatigue in advanced cancer – meaning before measurement? *International Journal of Nursing Studies* **37**, 401–414

Lanceley A (1995). Wider issues in pain management. *European Journal of Cancer Care* **4**, 153–157

Lanceley EA (1999). The patient and nurse in emotion talk and cancer. Unpublished PhD thesis, King's College, University of London

Lattimer V, Sassi F, George S *et al.* (2000). Cost analysis of nurse telephone consultation in out of hours primary care: evidence from a randomised controlled trial. *British Medical Journal* **320**, 1053–1057

McArdle JMC, George WD, McArdle CS *et al.* (1996). Psychological support for patients undergoing breast surgery: a randomised study. *British Medical Journal* **312**, 813–817

McMahon R & Pearson A (1991). *Nursing as Therapy*. London: Chapman & Hall

Mayor S (2000). Survey of patients shows that cancer pain still undertreated. *British Medical Journal* **321**, 1309

Middleton S & Roberts A (eds) (2000). *Integrated Care Pathways: A practical approach to implementation*. Oxford Butterworth Heinemann

Miettinen T, Tilvis RS, Karppi P *et al.* (1998). Why is pain relief of dying patients often unsuccessful? The relatives' perspectives. *Palliative Medicine* **12**, 429–435

Morris M (1996). Implementation of guidelines and paths in oncology. *Oncology* **10** (suppl 11), 123–129

Portenoy RK & Lesage P (1999). Management of cancer pain. *The Lancet* **353**, 1695–1700

Portenoy RK, Thaler HT, Kornblith AB *et al.* (1994). Symptom prevalence, characteristics and distress in a cancer population. *Quality of Life Research* **3**, 183–189

Preston N (1995). New strategies in the management of malignant ascites. *European Journal of Cancer Care* **4**, 178–183

Radley A (ed.) (1993). *Worlds of Illness: Biographical and cultural perspectives on health and disease*. London: Routledge

Riddell A & Fitch M (1997). Patients' knowledge of and attitudes toward the management of cancer pain. *Oncology Nursing Forum* **24**, 1775–1784

Rogers MS & Todd CJ (2000). The 'right kind' of pain: talking about symptoms in outpatient oncology consultations. *Palliative Medicine* **14**, 299–307

Rossiter D & Thompson AJ (1995). Introduction of integrated care pathways for patients with multiple sclerosis in an inpatient neurorehabilitation setting. *Disability and Rehabilitation* **17**, 443–448

Royal College of Radiologists (1998). *Interprofessional Roles and Responsibilities in a Radiology Service*. London: The Royal College of Radiologists

Saunders CM (1967). *The Management of Terminal Illness*. London: Hospital Medicine Publications

Scarry E (1985). *The Body in Pain: The making and unmaking of the world*. New York: Oxford University Press

Seers K & Carroll D (1998). Relaxation techniques for acute pain management: a systematic review. *Journal of Advanced Nursing* **27**, 466–475

Selwood K (2000). Integrated care pathways: an audit tool in paediatric oncology. *British Journal of Nursing* **9**, 34–38

Shum C, Humphreys A, Wheeler D *et al.* (2000). Nurse management of patients with minor illnesses in general practice: multicentre, randomised controlled trial. *British Medical Journal* **320**, 1038–1043

Sontag S (1991). *Illness as Metaphor/AIDS and its Metaphors*. London: Penguin

Stacey J (1997). *Teratologies: A cultural study of cancer*. London: Routledge

Stiggelbout AM, De Haes JCJM, Vree R *et al.* (1997). Follow up of colorectal cancer patients: quality of life and attitudes towards follow up. *British Journal of Cancer* **75**, 914–920

Sulch D & Kalra L (2000). Integrated care pathways in stroke management. *Age and Ageing* **29**, 349–352

Teoh N & Stjernsward J (1992). WHO cancer pain relief programme – ten years on. Newsletter International Association for the Study of Pain Seattle

Thomason TE, McCune S, Bernard SA *et al.* (1998). Cancer pain survey: patient-centred issues in control. *Journal of Pain and Symptom Management* **15**, 275–284

Venning P, Durie A, Roland M *et al.* (2000). Randomised controlled trial comparing cost effectiveness of general practitioners and nurse practitioners in primary care. *British Medical Journal* **320**, 1048–1053

World Health Organization (1990). *Cancer Pain Relief and Palliative Care*. Geneva: WHO

PART 6

Clinical education and the management of cancer pain

Chapter 12

Improving the understanding and effectiveness of cancer pain management through educational intervention: what exactly constitutes adequate undergraduate knowledge and how can continuity be maintained through postgraduate education?

Bee Wee and Richard Hillier

Introduction

In considering ways and means of improving understanding and effectiveness of cancer pain management, it seems perfectly reasonable to begin at the beginning, i.e. with undergraduate professional education.

What constitutes adequate undergraduate knowledge?

On consideration of a response to this question, it is perhaps useful to start by clarifying the intended endpoint. What is the aim of undergraduate education for health and social work professionals? We believe that a legitimate aim is 'to produce a competent and compassionate graduate capable of learning throughout his/her professional career'. This emphasises that the 'endpoint' of successful undergraduate education is only the starting point of the graduate's career and that undergraduate/ postgraduate education cannot be seen as separate; they are a continuum. In this chapter, we put up a mirror to this process. First, we discuss issues in modern-day undergraduate education, applying some educational concepts to our approach. We then move on to discuss postgraduate education. Finally, we address the issue of supporting the teachers within this educational process – something that is essential to the whole process.

In 1996, Coles stated that one of the tasks of undergraduate education for health professionals is to prepare students for their eventual practice. In the case of cancer pain management, preparing for practice requires much more than merely imbibing adequate knowledge. The requirements for undergraduate learning in cancer pain management are encapsulated in Table 12.1.

However, these requirements need to be maintained and developed throughout the individual's career and apply to all health professionals. Clearly, the depth to which these need to be understood, processed and attained will be commensurate with the

Table 12.1 A proposed 'core curriculum' for cancer pain management

Skills in assessment
Understanding of the role of analgesics and other drugs
Understanding of the role of non-pharmacological approaches
Clear and appropriate communication skills
A sound decision-making process
Critical thinking and action within an ethical framework

stage and level of experience of that individual professional and will differ for the different health and social work professional groups.

Case study: undergraduate medical education

There is little in the literature about the extent of undergraduate medical education in cancer pain management. The best evidence so far comes from Field's work (1984, 1995). Field (1984) first carried out a survey of medical schools in June 1983 enquiring into formal instruction about death and dying. At the time, only one of the 20 medical schools in the UK reported any teaching about pain relief at the pre-clinical stage. Six schools reported that pain management was taught at the clinical stage. A similar survey was carried out in 1994 (Field 1995). By this time, although only one of 21 medical schools reported that teaching about pain relief occurred at the pre-clinical stage, the number of schools teaching about pain relief at the clinical stage had risen to 23 (of 26 schools). Field is currently repeating this survey and responses so far (15 of 24 medical schools) suggest that students in all these schools get some exposure to teaching about analgesics for cancer or chronic pain (D Field 2000, personal communication). It must be emphasised that the primary focus of Field's studies has been the teaching of death, dying and bereavement; hence the data concerning cancer pain management education must be interpreted with some reservation. Nevertheless, it offers encouraging information about the increased teaching of pain relief within the undergraduate curriculum in the UK. What, however, do students actually need to know?

To ascertain what undergraduates need to learn about cancer pain management, we should consider the endpoint of their learning. One of the principal recommendations within the General Medical Council's (GMC 1993) publication *Tomorrow's Doctors* was that a core curriculum encompassing the essential knowledge, skills and appropriate attitudes that should be acquired at the time of graduation should be defined. In the 7 years since that publication, all medical schools in the UK have striven to define and implement core curricula. However, this task is rendered difficult because there is no nationally defined core curriculum and therefore each school has had to define its own, within its understanding of the GMC guidelines. There are no plans at present to develop a national core curriculum for undergraduate medical students.

However, if we accept the points in Table 12.1 as a core curriculum for undergraduate education on cancer pain management, we now have a basis on which to start discussions about the level of learning that is required, at which point(s) in the curriculum this learning should occur and who would most appropriately teach the students.

There are, broadly speaking, three main types of undergraduate medical curriculum in the UK, albeit with many variations on these themes. These are: the traditional pre-clinical/clinical curriculum, the systems-based integrated curriculum and problem-based learning. It is beyond the scope of this chapter to discuss the merits and problems of each type of curriculum; nor would it serve our purpose in trying to improve the understanding and effectiveness of cancer pain management through education. It is probably more helpful to accept the 'core curriculum' in Table 12.1 (warts and all) and translate this into the curriculum of our respective medical schools. To do so, we may usefully adopt some of the concepts promoted by our educationalist colleagues, who have made a huge contribution to undergraduate learning and teaching.

Applying educational concepts to cancer pain education

It is inappropriate in this chapter to discuss educational concepts in great detail. What follows are simply the thoughts of two clinicians with an interest in education and educational concepts that have proved helpful for the authors. We consider the issues surrounding the curriculum, how students learn and a little on assessment and evaluation.

The curriculum

What is a curriculum? Coles (2000) suggests that the curriculum may be thought of as comprising at least three overlapping circles (Figure 12.1). The 'curriculum on paper' states the aims and intentions of the course, as perceived by the curriculum planners. Specific learning objectives or learning outcomes are set explicitly, so that teachers and students can be clear about the steps that are required in order to achieve the overall aim of the course, e.g. one learning objective in cancer pain management might be that, by the end of the course, students are able to select a suitable analgesic for pain relief and to explain why they have chosen that particular drug.

The 'curriculum in action' is what happens when the paper curriculum is implemented. Some of this day-to-day teaching may have had explicit intentions (as in the curriculum on paper); others simply happen without planning. Some of the intentions of the 'curriculum on paper' might not happen at all. An example of learning 'simply happening' might be as follows. Although the role of newer analgesics might not have been a specific learning objective (perhaps because there is currently an inadequate evidence base for their use), students may hear about the existence of such drugs as potential analgesics of the future, simply by having a conversation with the teacher at the end of the session.

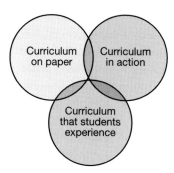

Figure 12.1 The curriculum (Coles 2000).

The third overlapping circle is the 'curriculum that students experience'. This is the learning that is actually picked up by students. Some of this learning was the explicit intention of the 'curriculum on paper'. Some learning happened as a result of either explicit or implicit messages that the teachers sent out, even though this was not an explicit aim of the curriculum planners, and some learning simply happened to form a part of the students' experience. This can have surprising consequences. Teachers need to be very careful of this. Enthusiasm, which is vital to all good teaching, can on occasions have negative effects, e.g. if students find that some teachers respond more positively to them when they discuss new analgesics, they may perceive the knowledge of new analgesics to be of more value than any other aspect of pain management.

Much attention is paid to the 'curriculum on paper'. The GMC and many medical schools have attempted to define a core curriculum for medical undergraduate education. More specifically, many specialities, including palliative medicine, have attempted to define the learning that is required for its particular speciality. However, Coles' model above demonstrates that attention must be paid to understanding the other two types of 'curriculum' (curriculum in action and curriculum that students experience), because they have a very powerful influence on student learning.

How students learn

Just as there are different aspects to a curriculum, so there are different types of student and student learning. Students can adopt a deep or surface approach to learning (Gibbs 1992). With the former, they attempt to understand the meaning of what they are studying whereas, with a surface approach, they are merely reproducing what they learn – the old concept, still occurring in some parts of the world, known as learning by rote. In terms of learning about cancer pain management, students adopting a surface approach may very well be able to reel off the commonly used analgesics, but may not be able to explain the rationale behind their use. However, only having a deep approach to learning is also insufficient for the management of cancer pain. The ability to explain the physiological and pharmacological rationale for using certain analgesics is only one part of effective cancer pain management. On its own, this might mean that the student has a clear understanding of the analgesics and of why, and when, they should be used.

However, health and social work professionals have to practise in uncertain and highly variable situations and environments, primarily because they deal with human beings who are both complex and unique.

A further process that seems to be required for successful learning in health and social work professionals is the process of elaboration (Coles 1990). This is where students see things 'fitting together' and find that knowledge gained in one area could be applied in others, e.g. having understood the range and applications of analgesics, they then discover that adding this to their skills in assessing the patient with pain enables them to apply that knowledge of analgesics in a more effective way, which in turn leads to better pain management. Students will also draw on their communication skills to obtain a relevant history and to discuss with and explain options and the management plan clearly to the patient. Teachers can assist novice students in this process by drawing the links to their attention, and by encouraging them continually to form further links through questions and discussions.

Experiential learning and reflection

Kolb (1984) suggests that learning occurs best when it is based on the learner's own experience. If students have the opportunity to reflect on their concrete experience, they are then able to consider what they thought and why they behaved or reacted in a particular way. These 'theories' can then be applied to a new situation, which provides further opportunities for experience, reflection and learning, e.g. having met a patient with pain, the student assesses the situation, considers the management options and proposes a particular course of action. Reflection on this process enables the student to explore his or her process of decision-making at the bedside, as described by Hillier (2000). It should then be possible to refine this next time the student encounters a similar situation.

However, there are problems for students learning in a modern National Health Service. Changing patterns of health care have imposed a change in teaching approaches. Acute hospitals now experience a more rapid turnover of inpatients and a move towards more day-case work, both resulting in a more transient and less stable patient population from whom the students may have to learn. Community teams now have to cope with patients who have more complex problems and who are being discharged from hospitals earlier than they once were. This results in a more acute and heavier case-load, again making it more difficult to organise teaching. Yet, patients must remain a powerful source of learning for health and social work professionals, so innovative approaches to learning are required. At the Countess

Mountbatten House in Southampton, lay carers are involved in the educational process within undergraduate interprofessional workshops (Turner *et al.* 2000). This enhances the authenticity of the students' learning experience by hearing the story (of the care received) directly from those at the receiving end, and creates the opportunity for students from several professional groups (medical, nursing, physiotherapy, occupational therapy and social work) to learn from, and with, each other. The carers also report positively on their experience and appreciate the opportunity to contribute to professional education.

Assessment and evaluation

Some aspects of the process of cancer pain management are more easily observable than others. The teacher can directly observe the student taking a history, examining the patient and communicating with the patient. The teacher is thus in a position to offer feedback and to help the student identify areas for further development – this is sometimes called 'formative assessment'. The teacher can also assist the student with the process of reflection through the use of 'whys' and 'hows'.

'Summative assessment' is different but has a profound influence on learning. The method of assessment used must be linked to the learning objectives set in the first place, e.g. if the learning objective is to know the range of analgesics available and to understand the rationale for using specific analgesics, then an assessment method that aims at measuring the number of analgesics known to the student simply encourages students to adopt a surface learning approach, in order to maximise their potential for passing the assessment. On the other hand, a case scenario or real-life situation that requires students to explain their choice of a specific pain management approach will encourage students to adopt a deep learning approach and to use Coles' (2000) elaboration in their learning.

It is important that students share ownership of their teaching and learning. They need opportunities to evaluate the teaching and to feed back in a constructive manner. If this opportunity does not exist, students will express their views in other ways, often less constructive, such as by disruption or simply 'not turning up'.

Postgraduate education

At the beginning of this chapter we emphasised that there is a continuum from undergraduate education to postgraduate education and personal development. After all we spend more of our lives as qualified practitioners than as undergraduate students.

All the concepts discussed so far for undergraduates apply equally in postgraduate education. However, there are specific challenges for postgraduate education that can be more difficult. These include problems with 'protected time', funding, conflicting demands on educational time, the rapidly changing patterns of health care, the frequent emergence of new drugs with new indications, interminable paperwork, and the struggle to fulfil every professional's continuing professional development needs within a busy workplace.

As a result of this, a range of educational formats is required to meet the varying learning needs and opportunities of postgraduate health and social work professionals. Some require formal direct contact or distance-learning courses; others cope better with single-day or lunchtime sessions; others feel they barely have time to stop. The only way to reach this last group might be to maximise opportunities for them to learn informally by observation, feedback and reflection within the work place. The development of a learning plan and guidance on how to achieve it may also be needed.

A distinction also needs to be made between education and training. Eraut (1994) cites Oakeshott (1962), following Aristotle, in talking about the difference between 'technical knowledge' and 'practical knowledge'. 'Technical knowledge' is easy to codify and convey to health professionals. 'Practical knowledge', however, is learned only through experience in practice. Professional judgement in health care is an example of practical knowledge, where judgements and decisions have to be made in real-world practice where uncertainty often lurks and where guidelines and protocols become less straightforward to apply than they may seem in theory. Tyreman (2000) explores the notion of the 'expert' health practitioner sometimes having to make the *best*, rather than the technically *right*, decision, where best equates to good (or most appropriate for that particular situation) and right equates to correct in the sense of the true or the approved (e.g. as in protocols and guidelines). He argues that this capacity for critical thinking is one of the key factors that differentiates the expert from the novice practitioner.

In considering cancer pain education in the postgraduate phase, therefore, the focus needs to shift to 'practical knowledge', using the learners' everyday experiences, both in uniprofessional and in interprofessional learning contexts. This not only makes the learning relevant and meaningful to the learner, it is also economical in terms of time and energy spent on developing learning materials.

Supporting the teachers

In this chapter so far, we have discussed the subject, the learners, the context and the learning processes. However, there is another critical factor in consideration of how educational intervention can be used to improve the understanding and effectiveness of cancer pain management – the teachers.

These teachers may come from a variety of backgrounds – basic scientists, clinical pharmacologists, palliative medicine specialists, pain anaesthetists, complementary therapists, primary care teams, etc., as well as other healthcare professionals. Most of these teachers have never been formally taught to teach. For many, teaching is not the prime focus of their responsibilities. If they are to become effective teachers, they need to be supported. To achieve this, the curriculum should be realistic and learning objectives clear. Initially, these 'teachers' need to teach within their 'comfort zone' – they should not be asked to take on teaching for which they feel unprepared. Some of the tips that might usefully be passed on to potential teachers are listed in Table 12.2.

Table 12.2 Getting started in teaching

Grab the opportunities
Consider the learner's starting point
Negotiate direction and destination
Ensure relevance
Provide hooks and 'stuff' (learning materials)
Enjoy it!

Many new teachers feel the need to attend teaching courses. However, before they do so, they should be encouraged to think through their learning needs (Millard 2000). Some of the questions they might wish to ask themselves are listed in Table 12.3. They may then choose to use peer observation, with structured feedback, as a powerful tool to help them to improve their teaching continually. Teachers will also need help to evaluate their own teaching, to develop the appropriate assessment tools and to invite and deal with feedback from students, whether positive or negative. A strategy for supporting the teachers has to be a fundamental part of any learning organisation.

Table 12.3 Areas for development: questions teachers might ask themselves

What is it that I want to be able to do differently?
Do I need more knowledge about the learning process?
Do I need to know more about the techniques and methods of teaching?
Do I need to examine the way in which I view my teaching and, maybe, change this?
Are my problems in teaching mainly organisational? For example, too few patients on the ward who are suitable for my students to learn from, or lack of a reasonable room in which to run an interactive small group session
Do I need to gain feedback about how I am doing as a teacher?
Do I need more practice in certain areas, such as writing learning objectives or producing a lecture at a suitable level for first year undergraduates?

Source: Millard (2000).

Conclusions/recommendations

If our overall aim is that all patients with cancer pain should receive effective pain management, then effective educational interventions are essential. These do not have to be sophisticated, but must be underpinned by sound principles, such as clear aims and objectives, appropriate teaching, learning and assessment methods, and a strategy for developing and supporting the teachers.

Within the undergraduate curriculum, learning opportunities are more structured and the use of a core curriculum, as in Table 12.1, helps to keep the learning and teaching focused. For postgraduates, teaching and learning opportunities are less structured and opportunities may need to be grabbed as they arise. Students are more easily motivated if they see the relevance of what they are learning. For some, this motivation will be the potential for improved patient care; for others, it will be the potential for passing the next examination! As long as they are provided with a clear framework for learning (rather like coat hooks), they will be able to organise their learning (the 'stuff' that hangs on coat hooks), so that they can easily access this learning when needed. The more opportunities there are for gaining concrete experiences and for reflecting on them, the more students will learn. All that then remains is for students and teachers to enjoy it!

References

Coles CR (1990). Elaborated learning in undergraduate medical education. *Medical Education* **24**, 14–22

Coles C (1996). Undergraduate education and palliative care. *Palliative Medicine* **10**, 93–98

Coles C (2000). How students learn. In Jolly B & Rees L (eds) *Medical Education in the Millennium*. New York: Oxford University Press, pp 63–82

Eraut M (1994). *Developing Professional Knowledge and Competence.* London: Flamer Press

Field D (1984). Formal instruction in United Kingdom medical schools about death and dying. *Medical Education* **18**, 429–434

Field D (1995). Education for palliative care: formal education about death, dying and bereavement in UK medical schools in 1983 and 1994. *Medical Education* **29**, 414–419

General Medical Council (1993). *Tomorrow's Doctors: Recommendations on undergraduate medical education*. London: General Medical Council

Gibbs G (1992). The nature of quality in learning. In: *Improving the Quality of Student Learning*. Bristol: Technical and Educational Services Ltd, pp 2–11

Hillier R (2000). Decision making at the bedside. What constitutes 'best medical practice' in the management of cancer pain? In Hillier R, Finlay I, Welsh J, Miles A (eds) *The Effective Management of Cancer Pain*. London: Aesculapius Medical Press, pp 25–30

Kolb DA (1984). *Experiential Learning: Experience as a source of learning and development.* Englewood Cliffs, NJ: Prentice Hall

Millard L (2000). Teaching the teachers: ways of improving teaching and identifying areas for development. *Annals of the Rheumatic Diseases* **59**, 760–764

Turner P, Sheldon F, Coles C *et al.* (2000). Listening to and learning from the family carer's story: an innovative approach in interprofessional education. *Journal of Interprofessional Care* **14**, 387–395

Tyreman S (2000). Promoting critical thinking in health care: Phronesis and criticality. *Medicine, Health Care and Philosophy* **3**, 117–124

Index

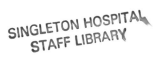